DEDICATION

This book is dedicated to my parents Abd
Almajeed Batterjee and Anne C. Schaerer-Batterjee.

A Fading

ART

Understanding Breast-Feeding in the Middle East

DR. MODIA BATTERJEE

ISBN: 1451542054
ISBN-13: 9781451542059
LCCN: 2010903548

ACKNOWLEDGMENTS

I would like to acknowledge the following people for their continuous support and patience during this challenging project: Khalid, my beloved husband; Omar, Maryam, and Eisa, my beautiful children; and Toni Williams, my editor. Finally, a special thanks to Reem Seraj and Maha Abbar who translated, transcribed, and helped me make sense of all the research data.

I personally find it fascinating that it was so easy for Saudi society to jump on the infant formula bandwagon. Sadly, they abandoned the best and most natural form of feeding their babies without even looking back. Every single day I hear the excuse about how slowly things must change here because people need time to get used to the change, for example, the idea of women driving, or of other social reforms. Why is it that infant formula was so readily accepted when there is so much information available about how much better, in so many ways, breastfeeding is for babies and their mothers? I just don't get it! Every single species of mammal on Earth breastfeeds their babies—yet Saudis are so easily convinced that it isn't enough, isn't good enough, and that formula is better? How in the world do they think that civilization ever managed to survive in the thousands of years prior to the introduction of infant formula? It just makes no sense!

Susie Khalil
Blog Author
Susie's Big Adventure, An American Woman moves to Saudi Arabia

CONTENTS

THE BEGINNING BY ANNE C. BATTERJEE

❧

Mothers are bombarded with statements related to breastfeeding benefits. Breastfed babies are protected from ailments including diarrhea, respiratory infections, otitis media, asthma, and many others. Additionally, WHO/UNICEF estimates annual deaths of 1.5 million infants worldwide because they are subjected to diseases related to not being breastfed. Somehow, we feel distanced from such horrors and perhaps a bit bored with the rhetoric. However, the awful truth is that infants in the Kingdom of Saudi Arabia are not immune to the negative consequences of bottle feeding, and our breastfeeding rates are not up to what they should be.

Since 1994, my public involvement in the "breast-feeding movement" has grown ever more active. Often as I stand in front of a group or auditorium filled with people waiting for me to speak, I think about what brought me to this point. I had always thought of myself a very reserved individual, and certainly not one to voice my opinion publicly. I had always preferred to stand back and listen to a debate rather than jump into the confrontation. Now I find myself easily flipping into lecture mode at any opportunity.

The reason behind this is probably due to the fact that I have been a victim of misinformation at some points of being a mother trying to nurture my child; yet, at other times of desperation, I was blessed with the knowledge and the support that allowed me to succeed. Thus, having experienced both failure and success, I feel very strongly the need to help other women experience the joys of success and help them to avoid the pain of failure and the consequences that may accompany it.

Motherhood began for me on October 27, 1970 in California. I was a very young mother, worried about my infant's health; I was alone and far from family and friends. My mother had breastfed all five of her children; she made it look so easy and natural that I had never even discussed the issue with her. So, young and alone, I faced my first child. The only thing about that experience that has stayed firmly in my mind is the calm gentle voice of the woman lying in the hospital bed to my right. Her voice was always there at the very moments I felt panic rise, telling me only just as much as I needed to know. She coached, supported, and guided me through those hard first days and nights in the hospital. I never knew who she was other than she was a La Leche League Leader and that she made a huge impact on my ability to mother my children. Her gifts of support and good advice have never dimmed. I have pursued every means within my reach to connect with La Leche League International (LLLI) ever since then, with the hopes of being able to pass on her support to every mother I meet.

Each birth brought with it a new and challenging situation. The healthcare system in most countries is not supportive, and trying to find those who could make positive suggestions is difficult because they are few and far between. That held particularly true for me as I settled into life as a foreigner married to a Saudi in Saudi Arabia.

Throughout the years, I knew that I needed to find a way to reach LLLI. In the late 1970s, long distance phone calls were still not an easy possibility. In a country where women do not drive, getting out and about is an issue. Over the next years, I heard rumors of the presence of nine different LLLI leaders who came to the Kingdom. By the time I found them, they were usually gone or at the end of their time here. Of course, all were "foreigners" and, therefore, lived in camps or compounds separated from the *local* world in which I lived. Each time I would hear the same story of how LLLI did not work here because of the living circumstances, which is quite understandable. At the same time, the Kingdom was plunging into the oil boom. Women were anxious to be "modern" and formula manufacturers saw the prospect of making billions in this unprotected developing market.

My frustration and determination has taken me on a long journey to try to bring not only LLLI presence to the women of this region, but to find a means of developing awareness and empowering women. In 1989, I suddenly found myself surrounded with women suffering from breast cancer. My father, a physician, said that statistically each of us should know four people with cancer in our lifetime. I had five friends and a sister-in-law all diagnosed in one year. Two of them had been breastfeeding, and had been told by physicians that the lumps were only blocked milk ducts. All five died within the next two years, leaving bewildered husbands and little ones behind. I knew something had to be done to empower women with enough knowledge to fight for themselves and understand their health care options. A hand full of women including myself started a cancer society; thirteen years later, I was happy to be involved in seeing it through to become a national organization.

In April 1994, an article in the local paper caught my eye. A prominent OB-GYN had written an article about the sad state of affairs of breastfeeding in Saudi Arabia. I was shocked to see that he felt that less than 20 percent of his patients breastfeed at all, but I knew he was right. At about the same time, an Egyptian doctor introduced me to the WHO/UNICEF Baby Friendly Hospital Initiative (BFHI), a program I could get my teeth into to make a difference! It took me over a year to convenience the government authorities that I should be trained. The fact that I was from the private sector went against the system, but in the end, I won. The BFHI national coordinator himself finally trained me as a BFHI breastfeeding counselor and trainer. I finally felt I had the use of a tool to improve health and to save lives by teaching mothers how to breastfeed their babies.

Breastfeeding is so much more than simply placing a baby on his mother's breast to feed.

How a baby is nourished in the first years of life affects his health, emotional development, and general wellbeing for the rest of his life. Many research studies on early development have shown that infants need a protective and caring environment to enable them to thrive into healthy individuals. Not only is breastfeeding important for the benefits to the child, but should be focused on and considered an important aspect of disease prevention and economic stability, which are a concern to any healthcare system. Careful attention to maternity healthcare, newborn health and nutrition, and the support needed to create strong family units is time and money well spent; it leads to better health status and better economic status of the community. In particular, enabling mothers to make healthy and affordable choices through supportive healthcare systems strengthens and financially boosts any society.

On a day-to-day basis, there is evidence that Saudi Arabia is a bottle feeding culture. A desperate need exists to evaluate the present situation and follow a strategic plan to work toward reclaiming the culture of breastfeeding. In order for this plan to be successful, it needs to establish breastfeeding as the norm and reclaim the mother-infant nursing pair as a model of ideal motherhood. Health care workers and maternity facilities are essential players in this plan and, therefore, any program should start at the level of the health care system. As a whole, the healthcare system should be the ultimate source of information and support. Positive changes toward the practice of breastfeeding in maternity facilities and hospital environments are necessary to any major change in the society related to breastfeeding and mothering practices. A second indispensable element of the plan is prenatal education of mothers; this will help them manage and overcome obstacles and potential barriers to improve their ability to sustain breastfeeding despite any problems that may arise. Empowering women means to build confidence in their ability to nurture their infants. Ultimately, there is the need to establish easily accessible support services within the community.

From my experience with trying to create a strategic plan to improve breastfeeding in Saudi Arabia, I have found many barriers. These barriers range from the individual to the highest levels of authorities responsible for infant feeding. A major obstacle in achieving the cooperation of the community and the authorities to implement a plan of action lies with the strong involvement of infant formula importation in addition to the subsequent formula companies' involvements in the health care system. The World Health Organization gives guidelines in this regard with a recommendation NOT to collaborate with manufacturers and distributors of infant formulas. The 1996 World Health Assembly recognized that sponsorship and other financial support from the baby food industry could create a "conflict of interest" among medical professionals. In fact, sponsorship will always explicitly require something in return.

The sad truth evident around the world is that the baby food industry always tries to undermine breastfeeding in order to obtain commercial benefit at the cost of child health; whether it is subtle or overt. By sponsoring events, this industry finds a golden opportunity to influence medical professionals by distributing literature with unjustified and unscientific health claims. Consequently, participants go home with misleading messages detrimental to breastfeeding and child health and nutrition in general. There is a great deal of literature in medical journals about the dialogue amongst authorities in regard to the topic of sponsorship and its creation of conflict of interest amongst members of the medical profession. The evidence always shows that, ultimately, sponsorship affects patient care, especially child healthcare.

Formula companies also use medical events as an opportunity to promote their products. The baby food industry frequently sponsors medical scientific meetings and educational events. They pay for entertainment during the events and set up promotional booths where product displays are exhibited. Participants receive promotional materials and "free give-aways." In Saudi Arabia, I have found that the majority of health professionals are not aware of, or are unwilling to admit, the power of these subtle gifts and sponsorship. In fact, it is well documented that these gifts and sponsorships create an unconscious bias that they cannot control. Brand awareness is secured.

The members of organizing committees and the long list of speakers at medical and health care events are the very people that Saudi communities depend upon to sift through and deliver vital and important messages to other healthcare workers. The people of this country turn to and depend upon all of them to deliver a high level of medical care in all government facilities. Any acceptance of funds from formula manufacturers hinders an unbiased atmosphere where families are able to make informed healthy choices. Acceptance of funds and sponsorship by noted organizations fosters the use of the health care system as a promotional channel and places health care workers in situations of conflict of interest. In 1987, an international group of doctors developed the "Doctors Declaration for Breastfeeding," which stated that signatories "under all ordinary circumstances will not accept personal funding from an infant food company for purposes such as travel, research, or equipment."

The Custodian of the Two Holy Mosques, HRH King Abdullah has called for a stop to the terrible situation of poverty and lack of housing for the people of his Kingdom. The administrative offices of the Kingdom's hospitals can be an incredible tool for him in his fight against poverty. By supporting, protecting, and promoting breastfeeding, each family can make informed choices, enabling them to afford food security for their infants and the rest of their family, rather than spending as much as half of their income for formula and treatment for unnecessary illness related to unhealthy feeding. Any needed formula feeds should be purchased just as a medication would be, thus eliminating the unnecessary practice of non-essential use.

A Breastfeeding clinic should be established within each hospital to serve as the focal point of implementation of the "BFHI 10 Steps to Successful Breastfeeding." Breastfeeding clinics or offices should be designed to provide breastfeeding support material and information for in-patients and out-patients needing support, as well as for staff members. These offices should also operate as a teaching center, housing for course curriculum, as well as a reference library. In this way, Saudi hospitals will become the resource centers for direction and information related to any and all issues that may arise in regard to breastfeeding. Realizing the severity of the problem, many governmental authorities, including AlShoura in the Kingdom of Saudi Arabia, developed legislation to control the baby food industry through various versions of the Code of Marketing of Breastmilk Substitutes. In addition, the Custodian of the Two Holy Mosques, the late King Fahad, signed the Saudi version of the Code into law in September of 2004.

In view of the above, it is my hope that each reader of this book comes to appreciate the seriousness of the matter. The Saudi breastfeeding situation is just as delicate and desperate as it is in most other places in the world, perhaps even more so since it represents the heart of the Muslim world, which according to UNICEF is one of the hardest hit by childhood disaster. Malnutrition and high mortality affect Muslim children most, according to a report released by UNICEF in September 2005. Islamic states account for the world's highest child mortality rates, where 60 percent of children die from disease and malnutrition before their first birthday. Over 4.3 million Muslim children worldwide under the age of five die every year and over one-third suffer from persistent malnutrition (UNICEF).

Our children are dying in direct relation to the decline in breastfeeding, which could so easily provide food security for at least the first two years of their lives. The Custodian of the Two Holy Mosques, King Abdullah has called for a stop to the terrible situation of poverty and lack of housing for the people of his Kingdom. The Offices of the Ministry of Health can be an incredible tool for him in his fight against poverty. By supporting, protecting, and promoting breastfeeding each family can better afford to secure food for their infants and the rest of their family, rather than spend perhaps as much as half of their income for formula.

This book is an important element in the struggle to attain awareness for the importance of breastfeeding in the region. I hope readers come to realize the need to protect our infants, our families, and our community.

PROLOGUE

If you have read the previous section titled "The Beginning," you have met my mother. This woman is described by some as "an angel"; she is kind, giving, tolerant, and very strong. My mother was the energy behind my accomplishments and the power that fueled my passion for lactation advocacy. I have spent the past four years with my head in the books and my focus on helping the women of Saudi Arabia. I was an International Board Certified Lactation Consultant (IBCLC) studying for a doctorate degree in Health Administration; my dissertation was on the breastfeeding situation in Jeddah, Saudi Arabia. Together with my parents, we opened the first and only breastfeeding resource and women's awareness center in Saudi Arabia during the four years of my study. In the center, I provided breastfeeding counseling for postpartum mothers and prenatal breastfeeding education classes for expecting mothers and fathers. I aspired to create an awakening for breastfeeding in the Kingdom, especially in Jeddah. After becoming exhausted with the public sector, I shifted my attention and energy to the private sector. I approached my targeted audience through a business so that I could create a demand that would develop into a pull that would force the public sector to conform and provide appropriate breastfeeding services to the entire community. During the past eight years, I have learned a lot about communities and how they function. I learned a great deal about the breastfeeding situation in the Middle East, specifically in the Jeddah community. Jeddah is a unique society that conforms very easily to trends. It is a special place where personal decisions and social behavior are largely influenced by many external factors. The factors are mainly religion, the media, Hollywood, and upper-class crazes. These external factors create the internal trends.

Some may believe that because Saudi Arabia is an Islamic culture, breastfeeding is common, and others may believe that an Islamic culture may make it more difficult for a woman to breastfeed. The Islamic teachings are very adamant about the importance of breastfeeding and the need for the child to be breastfed and in close contact with the mother for the first two years of life. Here are the four versus (translated) from The Holy Quran that support the practice of breastfeeding in Islam.

2.233: The mothers shall give suck to their offspring for two whole years, if [you] desire to complete the term. But the father shall bear the cost of their food and clothing on equitable terms. No soul shall have a burden laid on it greater than it can bear. No mother shall be treated unfairly on account of her child. Nor father on account of his child, an heir shall be chargeable in the same way. If they both decide on weaning, by mutual consent, and after due consultation, there is no blame on them. If ye decide on a foster-mother for your offspring, there is no blame on you, provided ye pay (the mother) what ye offered, on equitable terms. But fear God and know that God sees well what ye do.

❧

65.006: Let the women live (in 'iddat) in the same style as ye live, according to your means: Annoy them not, so as to restrict them. And if they carry (life in their wombs), then spend (your substance) on them until they deliver their burden: and if they suckle your (offspring), give them their recompense: and take mutual counsel together, according to what is just and reasonable. And if ye find yourselves in difficulties, let another woman suckle (the child) on the (mother's) behalf.

❧

31.014: And We have enjoined on man (to be good) to his parents: in travail up on travail did his mother bear him, and in years twain was his weaning: (hear the command), "Show gratitude to Me and to thy parents: to Me is (thy final) Goal."

❧

46.015: We have enjoined on man kindness to his parents: In pain did his mother bear him, and in pain did she give him birth. The carrying of the (child) to his weaning is (a period of) thirty months. At length, when he reaches the age of full strength and attains forty years, he says, "O my Lord! Grant me that I may be grateful for Thy favour which Thou has bestowed upon me, and upon both my parents, and that I may work righteousness such as Thou mayest approve; and be gracious to me in my issue. Truly have I turned to Thee and truly do I bow (to Thee) in Islam."

INTRODUCTION

The introduction of artificial formula and infant feeding supplements has given mothers a choice on how to nourish their infants. The basis for women's decisions include biological factors such as breast tissue insufficiency causing the physical inability to produce enough milk, cultural factors such as whether other mothers within a demographic area prefer to breastfeed or use artificial formula, and personal decisions such as whether or not a woman has the time, patience, and perseverance to breastfeed. Several research studies indicate that increases in diseases such as diabetes, obesity, and autoimmune disorders are likely caused by a decrease in the practice of breastfeeding. Studies also reveal that these diseases extend beyond infancy and affect the overall health of a nation, as children with diseases grow into adults. A sample of twenty women between the ages of twenty-one and thirty-five living in Jeddah, Saudi Arabia, with infants between the ages of newborn and four months participated in my dissertation research study that focused on capturing information regarding the influences that lead mothers to choose alternate methods to breastfeeding. The findings showed that an explanation for a mother's choice not to breastfeed exclusively was that Saudi Arabian, and perhaps Middle Eastern, society accepts breastfeeding but does not provide adequate support for breastfeeding mothers. The conclusions of the research study were used as the premise of this book in hopes that the information might assist in improving the understanding of breastfeeding culturally and perhaps for future national campaigns focused on promoting changes in cultural attitudes toward breastfeeding with the goal of reducing the rates of morbidity and mortality among Saudi Arabians and other similar cultures.

The following short story is fictional and not based on any real people or true story. Any similarities to actual experiences are completely coincidental. The story depicts an average Middle Eastern family faced with the arrival of a new member and the interaction between the family members and the placement of roles.

THE POWER STRUGGLE

"What about Mohammad? Let's just give the baby a name that can be universal and accepted by all," Fahad recommended to his wife, who was thirty-nine weeks pregnant, while he stood in the doorway of the master bedroom after coming home from a long day at work.

"Assalamu Alikum," she responded quietly, "When did you get home? I didn't hear you come in."

"Wa Alaikum Alsalam," Fahad sighed with a tone of frustration, because he noticed that she was packing her bags.

Sarah looked over her shoulder and saw that Fahad seemed upset. "It should be the other way around, you say AssalmuAlikum first. I am the one at home, and you were the one who walked in—Islam 101!" Sarah responded to Fahad while trying to figure out his frustration in her mind.

Fahad tore the ghutrah and igal off his head, threw them on the bed, sat down on the plush chair in their bedroom, and took off his shoes. He didn't make any eye contact and he didn't say anything more. Sarah continued to have the conversation about the name Mohammad. "But that is such a common name nowadays. I want my son to be special. I want him to have

a strong name, one that is appropriate for a little boy
and for a man. Mohammad is nice, and it is the name
of our beloved prophet, but today, people name any-
one and everyone Mohammad—men on the street,
strangers, waiters, cleaners. I don't know; I have to
think about it. I should ask my parents. My father wants
us to name him Abdalaziz, and my mother wants us to
name him after her father, Khalid. You know how she
feels about my father not letting her name any of my
brothers after her father. My poor mother, she had
to name her boys after the men in my father's family,
so typical of her times. It would make her so happy,
Alhamdulillah…my husband is different, right? You
are going to let me name my son whatever name I
want, right? Well, we can decide on the name together. We're not going to name him Abdulrahman after
your father or Hassan after your grandfather, right?
You are a modern man, one who lets his wife participate in these personal decisions. I am so lucky."

Sarah placed her nightgown and robe in her suit-
case and reached for her feather slippers. Her pregnant belly was too big, so Fahad kindly pushed them
toward her and asked, "Are you really going to wear
those?"

"Yes, I have to. There are going to be so many guests
coming to see me and the baby in the hospital. I have
to look nice. I have arranged for the hairdresser to
do my hair soon after I deliver too," Sarah responded
with a smile.

"Why are you packing so many things, how long
do you plan on staying in the hospital?" Fahad asked,
already knowing the answer, but hoping he would get
a different response.

"Fahad, I already discussed this with you, Habeebi, you know that this is our tradition, and we can't change it. You know that my mother decided that it is a better idea for me to go to the hospital from her house and not from our home. After delivery, all the girls stay at their mothers' houses for the forty days. It's not like you and I know anything about babies; we can't do things on our own. What if the baby cries? I am going to be too tired and will need my mother's help. At least that is what all the women say. I've never had a baby, so I am going to need my mother's help."

"Sarah, are you telling me that I will be all alone for six weeks? That is a long time. What if I want to see the baby? What if I want to carry him, and get to know him? I can try to help you, and your mom can come here to help you if she wants," Fahad said with sadness in his voice.

"Fahad, khalas (enough), this is our tradition, and you have to abide by it. This is how it is here in Saudi. Where do you think you are, America? Didn't I already tell you that mama and my sisters invited their friends and family for dinner tonight? We are going to be working on the final preparations for all the décor, chocolates, and guest favors. We're not going to be the ones who change this tradition," Sarah responded harshly.

"Fine, go. But choosing the name will be mine. You have to leave something to me. He will be my son, bearer of my name! Oh, and don't forget to pack your books. You need to learn about breastfeeding, or is your mom going to do that for you too?" Fahad left the bedroom, sat on the living room couch, and turned on the TV. "Sarah! Tell Fatima (the maid) to prepare my dinner, I'm hungry."

A huge cloud of sadness floated over Sarah's head. She suddenly felt alone and lost. Sarah truly loved Fahad and did not want to hurt or upset him, but he just didn't understand the importance of her mother's role in her delivery. Besides, Sarah didn't want to embarrass her mother in front of friends and family by staying with her husband and resting at home during her last month of pregnancy. Her mother had repeatedly told her that she would need her help, that she might need to use formula because she might not have enough milk to breastfeed. Besides, her breasts were small, and she would not be able to carry the baby and address all his needs by herself.

"Sarah you are fragile and inexperienced and cannot endure the hardships of motherhood. I've had five babies myself, and I know how to prepare the soothing teas for the baby and special foods for you just like my mother did for me. You cannot do it alone. We will have a great time when you deliver, I am so excited!" Norah prepared her kitchenette with new bottles, teats, a sterilizer, and of course, the most probably needed artificial milk formula for the baby.

Labor started, and it started fast that night. Fahad saw Sarah suffering in pain with every contraction. He quickly jumped out of bed, got dressed, and threw Sarah's abaya on over her nightdress as she wobbled to the door. Sarah moaned and groaned in the car on the way to the hospital. "Ya Allah, I'm sorry I upset my husband. The pain is unbearable, I am sorry. Ya Allah, please stop the pain! Forgive me Fahad, forgive me," Sarah wept.

Eighteen hours later…"Sarah gave birth to a lovely baby boy this morning" Norah boasted to her friend over the phone. "No, I didn't attend the delivery, I waited outside. You know I couldn't handle seeing my beloved daughter in pain," Norah explained to her friend. They said their goodbyes and she hung up the phone. Sarah's father walked in the sitting room, and the proud grandfather asked his wife if she was going to the hospital soon, as it was almost five in the afternoon. Norah explained that she was waiting for the florist to send his driver to meet her at the hospital with the flower arrangements for the hospital room. Sarah's parents paid several thousands of riyals to ensure that her room was decorated well to receive the congratulating guests.

Sarah and Fahad were delighted that the delivery was over. Sarah was left in her hospital room to rest and remember her delivery experience. As soon as the baby was born, he was whisked off to the nursery to be weighed, bathed, and fed, only to be brought back to his mother upon her request. Most Middle Eastern mothers prefer for the baby to remain safe in the nursery so that the mothers can rest and visit with her congratulating friends and family. Not many women understand the importance of early initiation of breastfeeding or understand that it is essential to build up the immunity of the infant with colostrum in the first hours.

Fahad was being kind, especially after his wife so earnestly apologized for last night's comments and asked her what she would like to name their son. "Khalid" was her request, but his mood suddenly changed and he said, "In sha Allah (By the will of Allah)." Norah suddenly burst into the room with hugs, kisses, and smiles. She was so very happy and delighted at the birth of her first grandson. "Ma sha Allah, Fahad; I am so proud of you. You endured her screaming and pain, what a brave man to be attending your wife's delivery. These are the men of the modern day. Khalas ya habeebi; you go home and rest. Come and visit us when we are settled at home. I will take good care of her and the baby. Bye!" Fahad felt like he was being pushed out of the room, which he was, of course. *It is very common for the Middle Eastern mother to take charge of her daughter and the new baby and to play a major role in decision making about feeding, changing, bathing, and all other care routines that involve a baby.* Fahad was just thinking about the baby's name, but decided not to discuss the subject in front of his mother-in-law. Fahad smiled at Sarah and quietly walked away.

As soon as Fahad fastened his seatbelt, he called his best friend Mohammad. *It is very common for Arab men to have a best friend with whom they share their worries and from whom to seek advice.* "Salam! Give me your congrats, my wife delivered our son. Alhamdulillah he is well, and she is okay."

"Mabrook (congratulations), mabrook; should we say Abu Mohammad (father of Mohammad) or are you thinking of something else?" Mohammad was very happy for his friend.

"Wallah I don't know. I need to consult with my father because Sarah wants to name him Khalid after her mother's father and I'm not happy with that, because everybody will think that I am a weak husband. What do you think?"

"My friend, if that is the way it is, just go safe and name him Abdulrahman after your father. That is our tradition, and it always works for the best. Her family cannot argue with you, and your father will be very pleased. You will also maintain your position in the family that way. Otherwise, you are in a losing battle with her family for eternity."

Fahad knew Mohammad was right, so he made arrangements to register the baby's name as Abdulrahman as soon as possible. Sarah would be happy that the name is not Mohammad, and his parents would be very happy with his decision.

Sarah spent two days in hospital with her female family members and friends; they visited while drinking coffee and tea and snacked on dates, biscuits, and chocolate. Her hospital room was decorated lavishly with baby bottle shaped ornaments hanging from the ceiling over her bed, the door to her room had a large welcome baby boy sign on it with two large floor arrangements, and the tables were garnished with trays of ornate dishes filled with flowers, chocolate, dates, and biscuits. The women laughed and giggled over stories of births, marital relationships, schools, child-rearing practices, and parenthood. Sarah was happy to be the center of attention and was pleased that the nice nurses took good care of her son and fed him well in the nursery while she rested with her guests. This was her mother's recommendation. She would not want her son to be exposed to diseases and illnesses that the guests might have unexpectedly brought in with them to her hospital room, would she?

"It is much better for the baby, and this will give your body enough time for your milk to come in," Norah mistakenly advised. Fahad called a few times during Sarah's stay in hospital and asked about his son, not disclosing to Sarah what he had decided to name the baby and leaving it a surprise.

Sarah's first night at her mother's house was a disaster. She ached with exhaustion and didn't know what to do with this screaming stranger. He screamed all night as she tried to put him to the breast for his first feed. Her mother stood by closely and assured her that her milk still hadn't come in, and it would be best to give him formula to stop the crying and try again for the next feed. "But mama, the book said that I should feed him at the breast when he's hungry. I didn't get a chance to read the entire book, but it said something about feeding on demand. Mama, please let me try. He is hungry, and I want to try." *This panicked behavior is commonly seen in postpartum mothers. After the festivities are over and real life sets in, mothers realize that they have an interest in breastfeeding. Mothers such as Sarah may have purchased a few books and skimmed through them a few days before delivery.*

"My dear daughter, you just said it. He is hungry, you don't have enough milk yet, and your nipples are very small. Just let me feed him, and you can try again later. It is sinful to let him cry like this." Norah grabbed Abdulrahman out of his mother's arms and stuffed a full bottle of artificial milk in his tiny mouth as she sat down comfortably on the bed. This practice was familiar to her and she acted naturally, the same way she had after delivering her own children.

Sarah complained to her mother, "Mama, Fahad really wants me to breastfeed; he said that it is recommended in the Quran, I have to at least give it a try."

"My dear, of course you have to breastfeed because it is recommended in the Quran; however, it is bad enough that Fahad didn't let you choose the boy's name, and now you're going to let him tell you how to feed the baby? He is not a mother, and he doesn't know how hard it is. He would die if he heard this screaming. Anyway, you don't have milk yet. Believe me, I know. What do you want to feed the poor boy, air?!" *In the Middle East, most mothers get into a power struggle with their daughters' husbands. It is very frequent for the daughter/wife to be caught in the middle. This example also demonstrates how breastfeeding is encouraged in the Middle East, but not supported.*

The struggles went on. Three weeks after delivery, Sarah continued to struggle with breastfeeding baby Abdulrahman. Norah continued to struggle with Sarah over motherhood. And Fahad continued to struggle with the loneliness that fatherhood brought him. Abdulrahman needed to be on a sleep and feed schedule that all babies were customarily put on as newborns. According to his grandmother Norah, "This feed and sleep on demand jargon is not acceptable!" Norah was training Sarah well for motherhood, according to her own experience. She felt that she had the experience and she knew well that carrying and holding the baby too much would only cause him to be spoiled and more demanding. *Norah's role was not unusual. In the Middle East, grandmothers usually take their daughters in and train them on how to feed and care for their new babies. Some believe that these women live vicariously through their daughters during this time.* "My dear daughter, you already fed him, why is he crying again," Norah asked Sarah as she walked into the guest bedroom where Sarah and her baby had been staying for the past three weeks. Sarah was carrying a screaming Abdulrahman over her shoulder as tears ran down her face. "I don't know Mama, I just breastfed him and now he's screaming again. Do you think he wants the bottle and not my breast? When I was feeding him, he was biting me and it hurt so badly but I forced him and I tolerated the pain, just like you told me to do."

"Sarah?" Norah questioned, "What if you don't have enough milk. Maybe your breasts are too small to feed a healthy boy. Do you think maybe you are just like me and my sisters? We never had enough milk. Poor thing, I was hoping you would end up like your father's sisters and breastfeed for two years."

Sarah felt the cloud of misery settle itself heavily over her head. Norah based much of her advice on personal opinions and what she heard other women talk about in the community. It is not unusual for an Arab mother to impose her personal beliefs on her daughter without any proper training or scientific knowledge. These statements are common and are meant as insinuations to influence the daughter's own beliefs and thoughts about herself. "Mama, I have milk! Look! It is dripping down my clothes. My breasts are not that small, but when he is breastfeeding, he cries. The book says that you can't give a bottle if you want to breastfeed, because the baby might get nipple confusion. Maybe he has nipple confusion." Sarah didn't know enough to decide whether or not Abdulrahman was suffering from nipple confusion, although her intuition was correct.

"Sarah, please! Don't believe everything you read. He's only a baby, what does he know? How can he be confused? He doesn't even think. He knows that your breasts are no good and that is why he cries. Maybe your milk is salty, or too light, or it hurts his tummy. Here, let me have him, I prepared his bottle about an hour ago, the milk is not bad yet."

Many Arab families believe that babies don't have feelings or thoughts and that they are trainable and become accustomed to what the mother enforces on them. Families in the Middle East and similar cultures often blame the mother's milk for the failure of breastfeeding, and it is common to claim that a woman's milk is light, salty, or causes vomiting.

Norah grabbed Abdulrahman once again, settled with him on the bed, and gently placed the plastic nipple dripping with artificial formula milk into his mouth. The baby sucked and sucked, as he learned to do in the hospital nursery, until his little tummy was full and he calmly fell asleep. Sarah sat in the armchair across the room and wept; she held her full breasts with both hands and watched her milk stream down her skin, soaking her nightgown for another night. Sarah's instinct told her that she had to breastfeed, but her ignorance did not allow her. The maternal hormones flowed through Sarah's blood as she watched her baby sleep in his grandmother's arm. She had the urge to grab him away and run home with him, but the traditional role of respect and honor for her mother controlled her and forced her to keep quiet and give in to sadness and what was called the baby blues.

It was a few minutes past midnight, and Sarah woke up to a screaming baby. He screamed so loud and forcefully that she felt hysteria taking over her mind. Sarah held Abdulrahman in her arms and bounced him gently to calm him down, but the screaming went on. She sat down and gently pressed his mouth against her breast, but the screaming continued. Her milk flowed, but he turned his face and screamed. He tightened his tiny body and his face turned blue. She stood up and threw him over her shoulder to help relieve

him of a burp or gas trapped in his tiny tummy, but the
screaming continued. He screamed and screamed until the small tears flowed out of his eyes as he cried with
pain. One hour later, Sarah could no longer tolerate
the screaming. She asked herself, "Should I give him
medication? I heard my friends talking about a medication to calm the baby down. What was it? Where do
I get it from? I can't. I can't do this anymore." Sarah
picked up the phone and called Fahad. "Fahad, my
love, I'm sorry to call you so late in the night, are you
sleeping?"

"Sarah?" Fahad was startled. "What's wrong? Why is
he screaming like that?"

"Wallah (in God's name), I don't know, he's been
screaming for over an hour now! And I'm worried, I
don't know why."

"Where is your mother? Wake her up!"

"I can't. Poor thing, she has been taking care of
him all day. I want her to rest. Anyway, she will probably just give him a bottle. I feel like she doesn't want
me to breastfeed, but I feel bad about thinking that
way. Of course, she wants the best for me. Maybe I am
just like her and her sisters and I don't have enough
milk, but Fahad, wallah, the milk is pouring out onto
my clothes."

"Sarah, leave the breastfeeding now; try to make
him stop screaming. How can you stand it? I'm not
there and it is driving me crazy!"

"I can't, I've tried everything. Can you come over
and take him to the doctor with me?"

"Now? It is two o'clock in the morning! There is no
doctor clinic open now; we will have to take him to the
emergency room."

"No, no, khalas (it's ok), I'll try to give him a bottle of yansoon, maybe it will settle his tummy. I miss you."

"Me too; I'll come over after work. Bye." *Yansoon is an herbal tea made up of anise seeds and caraway seeds boiled in water with natural sugar to sweeten it; the drink is used to relieve colic in babies.*

Sarah looked at her screaming baby, his little face looked so stressed and miserable. She reached for the prepared bottle of herbal tea, a concoction of yansoon, caraway, and sugar. It was cold, so she placed it in the bottle warmer for a few minutes to make it warm. Abdulrahman gulped the warm tea down and continued to whine as he fell asleep. Sarah felt alone. It was a weird feeling of relief and sadness; her life had been changed forever. She had been looking forward to motherhood, but now she realized that it was not fun; it was exhausting, confusing, and scary. Now that Abdulrahman was quiet, Sarah changed his diaper and gave him his midnight feed. She offered her breast and he suckled happily while his mother held him, enduring the pain. Suddenly the world seemed bright, and happiness filled both their hearts.

Sarah did not realize that the artificial formula milk was causing her baby to suffer from gas and hard stool. She also did not know that the more she fed him from a bottle with an artificial teat, the more he would suffer from nipple confusion, the more she would suffer from cracked nipples, and the more likely he would be to reject her breast. Norah did not know that telling Sarah to feed her baby from the breast less frequently would mean Sarah would have less milk.

Fahad sat up in bed; he couldn't stop hearing the screams of his son over and over in his head. "I have to bring them home. It has been three weeks and I have no role in my son's life. Maybe if I held him I could keep him quiet. I'm his father; he is my son. I'll bring them home with me tomorrow after work. It has been too long. How do other couples do it? I swear that with the next baby, I am forcing Sarah to stay home with me," he said to himself.

Morning came quickly, but Sarah could not open her eyes when she heard her son screaming again the same way he did during the night. Norah rushed in. "What? What is going on? Poor, poor boy, have you been screaming all night?" Norah picked the baby up out of his crib and carried him out the door. "You stay with me," Norah whispered to the screaming baby, "let your mother sleep," and she closed the bedroom door. Sarah was relieved to be alone and left to sleep. She closed her eyes and felt her breasts throb with milk. The pressure eased as the milk dripped into the breast pads and she fell fast asleep.

Sarah awoke that afternoon with unbearable pressure in her breasts; the pain was excruciating. The skin of her breasts was tight and red. She walked into the bathroom and stared at herself in the mirror. Oh my God! I can't bear the pain. "Mama!!" Sarah's screams echoed down the halls.

Sarah and her mother spent the rest of the day applying hot compresses to the breasts in an attempt to relieve her pain. Norah's recommendation to Sarah was to rest her breasts and not give Abdulrahman any feeds directly from the breast, because her milk was now too much and may be infected. Sarah was relieved by her mother's advice for two reasons. First, it was validated by her mother that now she had *too* much milk, second, she could not bear the pain and pressure in her breast and was happy not breastfeed the baby. That afternoon, Abdulrahman was bottle fed all the breast-milk that Sarah was able to express with an electric pump in an attempt to lessen the abundant milk supply. However, without Sarah and Norah's knowledge, the hot compresses and pumping kept the blood flowing and increased the swelling of the breast and the production of milk, causing no relief for the pain. Sarah cried.

In the evening, Fahad came over to pick up Sarah and Abdulrahman to visit the pediatrician to discover the reason behind the baby's crying fits. Norah was reluctant to let Sarah go, but she did not want to fight with Fahad, as he seemed very determined to take them.

Sarah's breasts hurt as she watched the pediatrician check Abdulrahman. The baby screamed, which made her breasts fill up with milk and throb; her breasts were so engorged that they no longer dripped as they did before. This made Norah believe that Sarah's breasts were infected with mastitis. Sara asked the pediatrician, "Why is he screaming like that? He screamed for hours last night, and I didn't know what to do."

The doctor spoke with great confidence. "Maybe your milk is not satisfying him enough. He may need more than you can provide." His words did not go down well with Sarah, because she knew in her heart that she had plenty of milk, and the evidence was that her milk had been leaking through her clothes. She dared not explain to the doctor what was happening with her body, as it would be too embarrassing to describe to him her breasts and how they were full with milk. "I think you should try giving him a lactose-free artificial milk formula. This is a new kind that might ease his suffering," the pediatrician recommended. Sarah smiled politely and packed up her baby and his diaper bag. She and Fahad thanked the doctor and left the clinic.

In the car, Sarah cried. As soon as Fahad asked her why she was crying, she began to sob. Her feelings of fear, frustration, and confusion were out of control. "I don't understand why everybody thinks I don't have milk, or don't have enough milk, or that my milk might be the reason that Abdulrahman is crying. I want to be a good mother, but my mother always makes me feel like I don't know enough. I know that she has good intentions, but her statements are strong. I feel like she knows more than I do, which is true. I don't understand why Allah would create a mother's body to make milk, but then gives her a baby that cries all the time and is harmed by that exact milk! How can this be?"

"Sarah, my dear, don't be upset. Relax. Please don't cry. It is just a matter of time and you will be in our home and together we can do what is best for Abdulrahman. Just relax, and do what you think is best for the baby now. Listen to your mom, because she has experience, and breastfeed him every time that you can. If he cries and shows that he is still hungry after you breastfeed him, give him the bottle of the lactose-free milk. That way you are pleasing everyone—your mother, Allah, the doctor, and Abdulrahman." Fahad realized the pressure that Sarah was under, and he felt that he needed to give her culturally appropriate advice that would not confuse her further or cause any more distress. Sarah smiled and her shoulders dropped as she stared at her beautiful baby sleeping in her arms. *It is not customary for families to use car seats for children and infants in Saudi Arabia.*

Sarah and Fahad felt comfortable with their decision. *It is typical for a young couple to try to please everybody in their social circle.* Day by day, Sarah's frustration with her mother subsided, especially when she moved back to her home with Fahad. However, she still struggled with breastfeeding Abdulrahman. The only times she could breastfeed him without a screaming session was when he was asleep. On good nights, the baby suckled gently at her breast as if he was soothing himself on a pacifier. This was okay with Sarah because she felt that she was doing her best and she was feeding him despite her severe reduction in milk supply.

Sarah shared with her friends that she was still breastfeeding him at two months. Many smiled in disbelief and others scorned her about breast milk not being nutritious or satisfying enough for a two-month-old baby boy. She heard comments like, "Poor boy, he will not be full if you only breastfeed. I hope you are giving at least one feed a day of formula," "When you breastfeed you are tied down, and the baby does not sleep well at night," "How can you breastfeed? Your breasts are so small, I'm sure you don't have enough." These comments hurt Sarah, but confirmed what her mother had been telling her all along. Everybody was saying the same thing, so it must be true. Sarah breastfed Abdulrahman as much as she could, but by the age of four months, he went on a breast refusal strike and weaned himself.

Two months later, it was seven o'clock in the morning and Sarah hadn't slept yet. She was rocking

Abdulrahman as he lay in her lap half-awake. Fahad was at a loss and did not know what to do to help; this was the fourth time that his now six-month-old son had suffered from an ear infection in just a few weeks. "His temperature won't go down" Sarah said to Fahad with a weak and tired whisper. "As long as we are giving him the medications there is nothing we can do," Fahad responded to her quietly. The pediatrician's voice repeated over and over in Fahad's head. He could hear him explain that their son could suffer from chronic otitis media (ear infections) if they were not careful, and that would mean surgery to insert tubes in the eardrums to protect any potential hearing loss in the future. The doctor's voice was interrupted by a piercing wail coming from Abdulrahman. Fahad jumped and ran over to his baby and tried to calm him down, he continued to ask, "what can I give you to help?"

All parents strive to provide for their children the best opportunities for health, education, and wealth. However, some parents may not realize how valuable and influential the practice of effective breastfeeding is on a child's wellbeing. Unfortunately, in the Middle East breastfeeding is not cherished as an investment that deserves the time and attention. The short story demonstrates how breastfeeding is recommended in a Saudi community but it is not supported. In most cases even if a mother and father have every intention to breastfeed their child the surrounding environment does not support it therefore forcing it to fail.

A PERSPECTIVE ON THE MIDDLE EAST AND SAUDI ARABIA

◦✖◦

The Middle East grew enormously during the oil boom in the 1970s and 1980s. The massive increase in oil-related wealth brought about dramatic changes in less than one generation. During the time of enormous growth, Middle Eastern countries like Saudi Arabia expanded with businesses, investments, and consequently, changes in community attitudes and lifestyles. Multinational corporations found a new land of massive opportunity, as the new and emerging nations had not yet put rules and regulations in place to restrict and monitor imported products.

Advancement in many industries brought about new demands, such as the need for women to work; thus, mothers who were breastfeeding needed replacements for human milk. Companies that manufactured infant formula aggressively marketed their products, specifically in Saudi Arabia, uncontrolled until 2004 when the first legislation was signed into law. This legislation is a version of the International

Code of Marketing Breastmilk Substitutes.[164] Through unchecked advertising, sampling, and overall financial control of governmental entities, infant formula manufacturers changed local women's breastfeeding practices by introducing artificial formula into infants' diets.[118] Formula feeding became the norm. The manufacturers became so successful in displacing breastfeeding with formula feeding that the results could be seen not only in the decline of breastfeeding rates, but also in the overall increase of illnesses that are directly related to feeding methods in early life. According to Saudi researchers, the occurrence of diabetes,[1] hypertension,[56] and cancer[10] have dramatically increased in recent years. Within a very short time, Saudi Arabian society moved so far from a natural-feeding method that the skills needed for breastfeeding were no longer a part of the culture.

Social theories might explain the lost knowledge of the importance of breastfeeding.[66] Bandura's social learning theory indicates the modeling of feeding practices of other mothers highly influences a behavior such as breastfeeding.[19] External influences might encourage as well as discourage mothers from breastfeeding their infants. Giugliani wrote, "The human species is the only one among mammals in which breastfeeding and weaning are not governed only by instinct" [64]. Giugliani concluded that breastfeeding and weaning are learned behaviors that a woman internalizes from her environment.

Researchers have been examining the breastfeeding practices of Saudi women. According to Shawky and Abalkhail,[129] breastfeeding declines quickly within the first year of a child's life in Saudi Arabia. The most common reason cited in the literature for the early introduction of bottle-feeding is mothers perceive breast milk to be inadequate.[5] Fida and Al-Aama noted several reasons for switching from breastfeeding to formula feeding: 50 percent of the participants reported inadequate milk supply, 12.7 percent of the participants were working mothers, and 10 percent of the participants reported their lifestyles did not allow for breastfeeding.[60] A common reason given by mothers and physicians for the decline in breastfeeding Saudi Arabia is that the mothers produce an inadequate milk supply.[5;60;129] Many health professionals and mothers have accepted this reason as justification for feeding infants artificial formula.[5;60;129]

The WHO and UNICEF developed the Global Strategy for Infant and Young Child Feeding to revive the world's awareness on the impact of feeding practices on nutritional status, growth, development, health, and survival of infants and young children.[165] The basis of the strategy is the evidence of nutrition's worth in the early years of life and on the idea that suitable feeding practices are a part of achieving optimal health.[126] In 2004, WHO/UNICEF reported the "lack of breastfeeding—and especially lack of exclusive breastfeeding during the first half-year of life—are important risk factors for infant and childhood morbidity and mortality that are only compounded by inappropriate complementary feeding." The impact is lifelong, and affects school performance, productivity, and intellectual and social development.[30]

Recent studies indicated a growing concern for the decrease in breastfeeding in developing countries.[129] Ogbeide et al. concluded that partial breastfeeding (mixing both breastfeeding and artificial formula-feeding) is the most common method of infant feeding in Saudi Arabia.[108] No research indicates why partial breastfeeding is the most common method of infant feeding and if exclusive breastfeeding exists at all in Saudi Arabia. The problem is that women in Saudi Arabia do not exclusively (solely) breastfeed their infants, which might be related to many of the health issues in the Kingdom. The lack of exclusive breastfeeding leads to higher infant morbidity and higher incidences of health problems in Saudi Arabia.[20]

This book was written with the intention of high-lighting the reasons behind Saudi women's decisions not to exclusively breastfeed their infants. I conducted a qualitative research study prior to writing this book, and the research results are used to describe the phenomenon of breastfeeding in Saudi Arabia.

An Overview of the Study

Data collection occurred during questionnaire-based interviews with twenty women from the city of Jeddah in the western province of the Kingdom of Saudi Arabia. Women were in the age range of twenty-one to thirty-five years, and had infants aged newborn to four months. The study provided data that might aid in understanding the phenomenon of increased formula feeding and in developing health improvement policies that protect, support, and promote breastfeeding. The findings concluded that breastfeeding in Saudi Arabia is accepted but not supported, and that the most negative influences on a new mother are: the lack of knowledge, the older female family members including her mother, hospital discouragement, and the social and cultural pressures against breastfeeding. This could potentially create a focus for the design of a national breastfeeding campaign and provide information that might help encourage necessary changes in hospital practices to facilitate breastfeeding Kingdom-wide.

The goal of the study was to provide descriptive data that demonstrates the need for prenatal breastfeeding education and to make available scientific data that support the revision of maternity protection laws and the creation of mother- and baby-friendly workplaces.

The "Innocenti Declaration," adopted in 1990 by the
WHO and UNICEF to protect, promote, and support
breastfeeding, urges all governments to develop national breastfeeding policies and set appropriate national targets.[82] The WHO and UNICEF also issued international guidelines for governments to establish a
national system that monitors the accomplishment of
set targets and the development of support programs
to improve the prevalence of exclusively breastfed infants at hospital discharge.[99]

Despite the programs and efforts in place, culture
and religion still have a significant role in breastfeeding. Saudi Arabia is an Islamic country in which the legislation derives from the Quran, The Holy Book, and
from Sunnah (also referred to as Hadith—teachings
of Prophet Mohammad). Religion has existed in every
civilization throughout history and commonly focuses
on the spiritual development of individuals, societies,
and cultures.[79] Khavari contended that religions have
basic features, such as a clear set of statements about
right and wrong and expectations for followers.[79]

As noted at the beginning of the book, Islamic law
requires all mothers to breastfeed their infants for the
first two years of life.[72] The law also requires the father
or heirs to support the nursing mother by providing
her with food and clothing throughout the breastfeeding period. If the mother is unable to breastfeed, the
father or heirs are required to provide another lactating woman to feed the infant.[72] The WHO, UNICEF,
Holy Quran, and Sunnah clearly state mothers shall
give suck to their offspring for two complete years.
However, though most mothers in Saudi Arabia start
breastfeeding their infants after delivery, they cease
quickly and introduce supplemental feedings.[5]

The Sociology of Breastfeeding

Researchers have spent many years determining how community involvement contributes to individual behavior and achievement.[49] Improved self-esteem and community involvement seem to set in motion a chain of events that can transform a culture.[49] Bandura contended an individual's personality was a combination of the environment, his or her behavior, and his or her psychological processes.[19] Cognitive learning theorists believe human development is represented in the best form "as a continuous reciprocal interaction between children and their environments"[128] also known as reciprocal determinism. Reciprocal determinism is "the notion that the flow of influence between children and their environments is a two-way street; the environment might affect the child, but the child's behavior will also influence the environment"[128].

Bandura believed humans are beings of cognition, and theorized that humans are active information processors, which means that humans are aware of the relationships among their behaviors and understand the consequences of those behaviors.[19] Humans are also affected by what they perceive will happen rather than only by what they truly experience.[19] Observational learning is essential to the human developmental processes in Bandura's cognitive social learning theory. Bandura suggested that when an individual observes another behave in a specific way, he or she is able to replicate the behavior when put in the same situation later. Bandura called the phenomenon "observational learning" or "modeling," and called the theory "social learning theory."

According to Bandura,[19] a child learns new behaviors simply by observing the behavior of others.
Individuals in a child's environment are social models;
the child makes mental notes of the observed behavior and then uses the mental notes to reproduce the
social model's behavior at some point in the future.
Observational learning, according to Bandura, allows
young children to develop several new responses in a
variety of settings in which the social models simply
pursue their own activities and do not try to teach the
child anything.

As stated earlier, Giugliani noted that humans are
the only mammals in which breastfeeding and weaning
are not purely instinctive. Giugliani concluded breastfeeding and weaning must be learned; a mother must
have learned her feeding practices from a social model
in her environment, similar to what Bandura explained.
La Leche League International agreed with Giugliani's
statements and contended that breastfeeding is an art
passed on from one mother to another.[140] Cognitive social learning theory, Giugliani, and La Leche League
all help to clarify why Saudi women cease to breastfeed
their infants and introduce supplemental feedings.

Influences on Breastfeeding

The unquestioned acceptance of breastfeeding
as the optimal practice remains vague and unclear
throughout the developed world.[20] Behaviors, practices, and beliefs that mothers are exposed to highly
influence breastfeeding and infant-feeding choices;[103]
this was clearly demonstrated in the short story. Social
and global influences might encourage as well as dis-

courage mothers from breastfeeding their infants. The following is a discussion of environmental, commercial, marketing, and health-care influences that might have a role in mothers' decision making.

Social Influences

In modern societies, women have few opportunities to learn about breastfeeding because the more traditional sources of learning, such as older women in the family, were lost as nuclear families replaced extended families.[64;141] Mothers become mothers with almost no knowledge about breastfeeding, leaving them vulnerable to problems during the process.[64] Common problems in the early postpartum period, such as sore or cracked nipples, infant breast refusal, and engorgement usually result in breastfeeding cessation and the introduction of artificial feeding.[141] Regardless of recent scientific verification that artificial formula feeding is a detrimental practice,[13] women continue to choose to feed their infants with artificial formula.[98] Mothers of new infants in Saudi Arabia might practice what they observe other mothers doing, thus, changing the ancient learned skill of breastfeeding to modern partial breastfeeding in recent generations.

Many cultural practices create obstacles for the practice of exclusive breastfeeding.[103] The present dominance of artificial formula feeding is apparent in the accepted beliefs of women that artificial formula can be as good for infants if not better than breast milk.[17]

In reference to Bandura's cognitive social learning theory, it can be concluded that new mothers are influenced by other mothers in their nuclear families, who are social models. Therefore, the new mothers stop breastfeeding their infants and introduce supplemental feedings when suggested to do so.[19] Additionally, an appropriate assumption is that infant-feeding practices in a community are gained from a mother's surroundings, regardless of the religious value or scientific significance. The understanding of social learning theories allows one to infer that local feeding practices are a social practice that one mother models for another; the mothers together then change the environment from a breastfeeding culture to an artificial-feeding culture.

Environmental Influences

From an ecological perspective, Bronfenbrenner put forward that each individual develops within a context.[32] The ecological perspective is the most detailed approach and analysis of the environment. In an attempt to understand how individuals influence and are influenced by their environments, Bronfenbrenner developed the ecological model. The ecological model has a microsystem, a mesosystem, an exosystem, and a macrosystem.[32]

The microsystem is the most immediate and earliest mutual influence of the child, parents. The mesosystem is an intermediate level of links and interrelationships among microsystems, such as social institutions, schools, and peers. The exosystem includes settings that influence the development of a child without direct contact, such as a parent's workplace, social networks, and local government. The macrosystem, the most distant, consists of influences such as global changes and the broader culture.[32] Bronfenbrenner's ecological systems theory and model explains the context of development and provides an idea regarding how people create accepted behaviors in their mind by what they identify with in their own surroundings. A lactating mother might develop accepted lactation practices in her mind by what she knows from within her surroundings, by what she might express to her environment, and the environment's reaction to her behavior.

Commercial Marketing Influences

Chang noted that the method in which information is presented or framed has an influence on an individual's reasoning and decision-making abilities.[39] Positively framed concepts generate positive associations and are more attractive than negatively framed concepts.[39] Braun-Latour and Zaltman discussed two types of information that influence decision making: internal and external.[29] Internal information is information gained through life experiences, and external information is information an individual encounters that might influence his or her beliefs.[29]

Advertising is an external source of information with a goal to persuade; advertisers hope to influence consumers through exposure to an advertisement, therefore, turning an external influence into an internal one.[29] Braun-Latour and Zaltman reported, "Ideally, the advertising content moves from being considered an external source and has become integrated into the consumers' own internal knowledge system" (p. 58). Advertisements have an enduring emotional impact on consumers, and consumers adopt an advertising claim as their own. Greiner, Van Esterik, and Latham contended women's belief regarding insufficient milk is a fundamental reason given by mothers who terminated breastfeeding as an example of the impact of advertising.[67] Although many health-care experts are skeptical, some simply assume women cannot produce sufficient amounts of breast milk. A major implication of the assumption is the widespread necessity for a substitute for human milk, even in early infancy. The observation is highly attractive to artificial infant formula companies, who often stress the significance of insufficient milk in their documentations and advertisements, making it a commercially induced syndrome.[67]

Health-Care Influences

The medical community has become the reference and source from which to seek medical advice, with value set on physicians according to the quality of knowledge and skill they can bring to patients.[104] Nevertheless, the medical community might still lack the proper information to support and overcome common breastfeeding resistance due to lactation problems because schools of medicine, nutrition, nursing, and public health have failed to include breastfeeding education in their curricula.[120] Formula company advertisements have distracted healthcare professionals from seeking the appropriate information to maintain and sustain proper breastfeeding practices.[20] Health-care professionals have a very important role in supporting women to enable them to breastfeed and to convince them, when appropriate, that artificial breast milk substitutes are unnecessary.[120] In fact, the lack of knowledge and the aggressive advertising of formula companies to the medical community might have caused breastfeeding rates to decline.[20]

Summary of Influences

In summary, the behaviors, practices, and beliefs mothers are exposed to highly influence breastfeeding and infant-feeding choices.[103] Although sometimes it is easier to focus on family or community influences taking place in human development, other significant influences exist.[80] Social and global influences might encourage as well as discourage mothers from breastfeeding their infants. Giugliani proposed that health professionals play a critical part in the prevention and management of breastfeeding difficulties.[64] Health professionals are key individuals in the processes of human reproduction and nutrition. "Education is a key step in the acquisition of appropriate skills and attitudes relevant to the provision of healthcare"[61]. The key players should have proper and updated training for providing the best care, including breastfeeding promotion and management.[124]

The beliefs and values of other women, their families, the workplace, and the health professionals involved in their care, as well as formula milk advertisements, can strongly direct the decision to breastfeed. Core and early research indicates the norms and beliefs must be positively influenced and directed to proper infant-feeding practices that support, promote, and protect breastfeeding.[24] Studies on the determinants of the breastfeeding patterns of working women concluded stronger social and healthcare support of exclusive breastfeeding is necessary before the full impact of workplace support can be truly examined.[24;119] According to Rea, Venâncio, Batista, et al.,[119] the duration of exclusive breastfeeding in São Paulo, Brazil, was highly associated with socioeconomic variables such as occupation of the mother, presence of a housemaid, and delivery room practices. This might also be applicable to countries such as Saudi Arabia. The research conducted in Brazil showed results that demonstrated the median duration of exclusive breastfeeding, predominant breastfeeding, and any breastfeeding at all were ten, seventy, and 150 days, respectively; by one month, 86 percent of mothers gave their babies tea, 50 percent of mothers gave water, and 42 percent fed artificial formula milk. Why mothers increase alternative feeding to replace breast milk remains unclear. Rea, Venâncio, Batista, et al. indicated maternity ward routines were not supportive, and that women adjusted their feeding patterns based on their anticipation of support from the workplace.

Scientific evidence supports the practice of exclusively breastfeeding infants. Edmond et al. noted breastfeeding promotion is essential for any child survival strategy and should be practiced in all nations.[55] The community and the medical establishment should emphasize early initiation and exclusivity to ensure successful breastfeeding practices and the establishment of a sufficient milk supply.[55] Infants must learn to attach and suckle effectively at the breast during the first days of life to breastfeed successfully.[78] Promoting the early initiation of breastfeeding can make great contributions to child survival. Edmond et al. concluded that 16 percent of neonatal deaths could be prevented if newborns were breastfed from the first day and 22 percent could be prevented if newborns were breastfed within the first hour after birth. Weinberg noted breast milk is undoubtedly the best nutrition for infants.[149] Great efforts must be spent to ensure proper and appropriate infant-feeding practices. Wright, Bauer, Naylor, Sutcliffe, and Clark contended exclusive breastfeeding was an effective means of reducing infant illness at the community level.[167] A reduction in morbidity and mortality was strongly associated with breastfeeding,[71] making it important to understand why Saudi women practice partial breastfeeding with their infants.

The Medical Implications of Breastfeeding

The medical community commonly supports breastfeeding as the healthiest method to feed infants.[136] According to Kroeger and Smith,[88] breastfeeding is a normal continuum to the childbearing cycle. The WHO defined exclusive breastfeeding as when an infant is only fed human breast milk without any food or drink other than vitamins and minerals.[164] Initiation of breastfeeding is the estimated time when the first breastfeed begins, which is recommended to be within the first thirty to sixty minutes after birth.[55] Prelacteal feeding refers to when an infant receives water-based feeds, which include glucose water, teas, infusions, or infant formula milk before the first breastfeed.[136] Prelacteal feeds might be given for many reasons; in some communities, they are given for traditional and cultural causes believed to enhance a child's health and well-being. Many cultures withhold breastfeeding for up to forty-eight hours while giving prelacteal feeds.

Szajewska et al. noted predominant breastfeeding is a term that applies when the infant's primary source of nourishment is breast milk, but the infant might also receive water, water-based drinks, and ritual fluids such as herbal teas, ghee, or honey. Partial breastfeeding occurs when breastfeeding and supplemental formula-feeding are combined as the main feeding method for an infant.[165] With formula-feeding, an infant receives artificial baby milk, also known as formula. The concoction contains the same categories of nutrients as breast milk, but does not duplicate them.[148]

Step three of the "Ten Steps to Successful Breastfeeding" recommended by the WHO states all pregnant women should be informed about the benefits and management of breastfeeding.[148] In 1992, the Global Criteria for the WHO/UNICEF Baby Friendly Hospital Initiative (BFHI) recommended pregnant women of thirty-two weeks or more gestation should be able to confirm the benefits of breastfeeding were discussed with them and that they understand the importance of exclusive breastfeeding to their children and their own health. In Saudi Arabia, it is assumed by the community that breastfeeding is the norm because of the religious influence, but only one study has investigated the topic. The results of the study indicated only 27 percent of mothers exclusively breastfed and 66 percent partially breastfed in the Saudi Arabian community studied.[108]

Benefits of Breastfeeding

Much of the literature establishes exclusive breast-feeding as the ideal method of feeding infants.[124] Breastfeeding is critical for child survival and, according to medical research, no better way exists to secure the best start in life.[149] Scientific studies show infants "become more productive members of society as adults if their health and neurological potential are maximized through optimal nutrition and appropriate health care from the start"[15]. The American Academy of Pediatrics highly recommends mothers practice exclusive breastfeeding for the first six months after delivery.[138] WHO/UNICEF's BFHI recommends against feeding infants food or drinks besides breast milk unless medically indicated.[165] The Expert Consultation on Breastfeeding advocated the practice of exclusive breastfeeding by the mother for the first six months of life, with the introduction of complementary foods and continued breastfeeding from six months on.[162]

Scientific research strongly supports the benefits of exclusive breastfeeding for the first six months of life.[69;124] Breastfeeding presents the perfect nourishment for all infants because it contains all the nutrients, antibodies, immune factors, and antioxidants infants require to thrive.[126] Many years of research demonstrated the health and economic significance of breastfeeding for children, mothers, and society.[86;150] Weinberg reported the promotion of universal breastfeeding plays an important part in the enhancement of child health by supplying the finest nutrition, providing a defense against widespread childhood infections, and promoting child spacing.[149] Breastfeeding exclusively suppresses the hormones for ovulation, therefore, not allowing a mother to menstruate or ovulate during the first six weeks after delivery.[41] The suppression of monthly menstruation and risk for pregnancy maintains maternal health and well-being, which allows the family as a whole to better care for its children. A research study conducted to examine the effects of breastfeeding and birth spacing on childhood mortality clearly demonstrated the positive effects on infant survival.[41] The evidence indicated increased mortality risks are associated with closely spaced births.

Breastfeeding is the most complete form of nutrition, not only because it provides normal nutrition for infants, but also because it provides protection from a range of diseases for the mother and child.[86;150] Breast milk contains digestive enzymes that make digestion easy; essential vitamins, minerals, and hormones; and antibodies that destroy any microorganisms that might enter the stomach, providing protection against infection and disease.[72] The exceptional dietary contributions of breast milk include the most favorable amounts and variations of proteins, such as long-chain polyunsaturated fatty acids and nucleotides, carbohydrates, micronutrients, and pharmacologically active components.[92;149] Human breast milk contains a wealth of immunological factors, including the antibodies lysozyme, lactoferrin, neutrophils, macrophages, and lymphocytes. The humoral and cellular immonoactive substances directly relate to the significant protection of infants from gastrointestinal infections, lower respiratory infections, otitis media, and meningitis.[92;149] Breastfeeding protects infants and children from common ailments such as diarrhea and acute respiratory infections. Breastfeeding also has a role in decreased child morbidity and mortality.[84;149] The significant role of suitable breastfeeding practices in the survival of infants is clear.[71] The decline of deaths from acute respiratory infection revealed the widespread beneficial effect of exclusive breastfeeding in the prevention of infectious diseases beyond breastfeeding's role in nutrition and food contamination.[107]

Breast milk is produced daily depending on an infant's need for growth and nourishment, compared with artificial formula milk, which remains the same regardless of the daily requirements needed.[72;81] A good example is the excretion of colostrum in the first days after delivery. The yellowish milk is an exceptional liquid that contains protein, minerals, and antibodies that sustain the infant's health and boost immunity with a surge of antibodies that protect the infant from first-time exposure to many organisms.[72;81] Breastfeeding, specifically exclusive breastfeeding, plays an important role in reducing exposure to contaminated food and drink at such a young age, which contributes to strong protection against infection-related deaths in childhood.[84]

Breastfeeding relates directly to normal infant growth and development, both physically and intellectually.[30] Researchers have indicated breastfed infants had lower rates of bacterial infections, fewer allergies,[126] less obesity,[14;69] and lower risk for long-term diseases such as diabetes and hypertension.[96;112;135] Researchers of many peer-reviewed articles reported breastfeeding practices are a determinant of future health status.[111] Science has demonstrated that breastfeeding early in human life might protect an individual from many common diseases. In addition, breast milk is the physiological standard for human development.[70]

Owen et al. wrote an article on the effect of infant feeding on the risk of obesity, which indicated breastfeeding was a determinant of one's state of health.[111] Owen et al. also examined the influence of initial infant feeding on obesity in adulthood.[111] The results of the research demonstrated initial breastfeeding protected against obesity in the future. A second article by Owen et al. also supported breastfeeding as a determinant of future health status.[112] Owen et al. posited, "Observational evidence suggests that having been breastfed in infancy might reduce the prevalence of type 2 diabetes in later life"[112].

Martin et al. wrote an article on the subject of breastfeeding in infancy and blood pressure in later life. They concluded a small reduction of systolic and diastolic blood pressure was associated with being breastfed in infancy, which was a benefit to cardiovascular health at the population level over time.[96] Martin et al. recommended further understanding of the mechanisms underlying the association of breastfeeding and adult diseases. Understanding the importance of early breastfeeding might provide insight into future directions that connect early life exposures to health in adulthood.

Mortensen et al. conducted a study to determine the association between duration of breastfeeding and intelligence in adulthood.[100] Many researchers strongly suggest the presence of a positive association between breastfeeding duration and intelligence in early and middle childhood, but not many examined breastfeeding duration and intelligence in adulthood. Mortensen et al. reported the duration of breastfeeding related to significantly higher scores on verbal, performance, and full-scale Wechsler Adult Intelligence Scale IQs. Mortensen et al.'s results demonstrated IQs of 99.4, 101.7, 102.3, 106.0, and 104.0 for breastfeeding durations of one month, two to three months, four to six months, seven to nine months, and more than nine months, respectively. Mortensen et al. concluded, independent of a variety of possible confounding factors, a significant positive correlation existed between duration of breastfeeding and adult intelligence in two independent groups of young adults assessed with two different intelligence tests.

The act of breastfeeding is associated with improved glucose and insulin homeostasis in adulthood. In a study on duration of lactation and incidence of type-2 diabetes, Stuebe et al. reported longer durations of breastfeeding related to lower incidences of type-2 diabetes.[135] Stuebe et al. sought to evaluate the relationship between lactation history and the incidence of type-2 diabetes in mothers. The study was a prospective observational cohort study of 83,585 childbearing women in the Nurses' Health Study (NHS) and a retrospective observational cohort study of 73,418 childbearing women in the Nurses' Health Study II (NHS II). The main outcome measure was the occurrence of type-2 diabetes. The results indicated that for each additional year of breastfeeding, mothers who had given birth within the previous fifteen years had a 15 percent lower risk of diabetes among the NHS participants, and a 14 percent lower risk among the NHS II participants.

Body mass index (BMI) and other relevant risk factors were controlled for. Stuebe et al. concluded that breastfeeding might reduce the risk of type-2 diabetes in mothers by improving glucose homeostasis.

Health problems in children can relate directly to their environment and their feeding practices. During growth and development, children might be exposed to contaminants and agents that damage the morphology of the developing tissue, causing diseases and disorders ranging from learning disabilities to cancer.[144] The scientific community closely monitored cancer rates and noted it could be deduced that breastfeeding had a role in the reduction of cancer rates. Van Den Hazel et al. noted, "In order to improve prevention, breastfeeding longer than six months confers some protection against acute lymphoid leukemia and should be encouraged" (p. 22). The benefits are not limited to infants, and breastfeeding mothers might potentially benefit from improved health as well. According to Ursin et al.,[143] lactation was directly associated with a reduced risk of cancerous breast tumors in women. Labbok posited that breastfeeding could dramatically lower the risk of premenopausal breast cancer by 4.3 percent for every year of breastfeeding.[90] The Collaborative Group on Hormonal Factors in Breast Cancer supported Labbok's view.[45] In a Korean study,[97] the duration of breastfeeding was positively associated with a considerable reduction in breast cancer. Strong evidence existed that breastfeeding might be accountable for approximately two-thirds of estimated reductions in breast cancer incidence.[45]

Breastfeeding an infant into childhood has economic significances as well as health benefits. Bronston contended that breastfeeding is best for the baby and more affordable for the mother.[33] A mother who breastfeeds her infant does so at no cost to herself or her family; the milk is provided biologically with the perfect form and ideal temperature. Purchased bottles, teats, or sterilizing equipment are not necessary. A breastfeeding mother might also reap the economic benefits of fewer illnesses and fewer physician visits for her infant; hence, mothers who breastfeed their infants have lower health-care costs than mothers who formula feed.[117] The medical and economic value of breastfeeding is high because breastfeeding seems to result in cost savings for parents, insurers, employers, and society as a whole.[122]

For the first six months of a child's life, breastfeeding can provide wholesome, clean, pure, fresh feeds at optimal temperature with the perfect balance of proteins, carbohydrates, and micronutrients, including hormones and nucleotides.[109] Human breast milk provides a growing infant with its nutritional needs of long-chain polyunsaturated fatty acids for brain development. Breastfeeding protects against a multitude of environmental insults a brand-new infant has not been previously exposed to, allowing the immune system to mature without unnecessary premature stress.[109] Weinberg posited,[149] "These nutritional, anti-infective, and birth spacing advantages of breastmilk led to widespread recommendations to promote nearly universal breastfeeding" (p. 200).

To obtain the health and economic benefits related to breastfeeding, society must support breastfeeding promotion as a social responsibility.[131] Walker reported human milk is species-specific,[148] and Williams wrote,[151] "Milk made by human mothers [is] for human infants" (p. 1). Breast milk evolved throughout time to make possible the finest growth and development of human infants.[148] Although many mothers choose to formula feed or partially breastfeed their infants, they might not understand breast milk is exceptionally complex and its "composition is most likely programmed by chemical communication between the mother and the infant"[148].

Hazards of Prelacteal Feeds and Partial Breastfeeding

Many studies revealed findings demonstrating differences in nutritional status between breastfed and bottle-fed infants in the developing world.[22;125] Exclusive breastfeeding in the first year of life could reduce the number of children worldwide who die from malnutrition under the age of five years.[25] Supplemental feeding, whether by cup or bottle, has detrimental effects on breastfeeding duration and infant health.[54;78] Prelacteal feeds and partial breastfeeding are not recommended, and the latter has been associated with a high-risk rate of infant death as a result of infectious disease.[54] The WHO/UNICEF's BFHI contend that the practice of prelacteal feeds or partial breastfeeding might delay the onset of full breast milk production or influence early termination of breastfeeding and early weaning of the infant.[165] Howard et al. indicated supplemental formula feeding had a strong association with the early termination of breastfeeding. Edmond et al. established that partially breastfed infants were six times more likely to have a higher mortality rate risk from infections than exclusively breastfed infants.[54] Exclusive breastfeeding is the ideal feeding method during the first six months, and then complementary foods can help meet growing infants' nutrient requirements.[41]

Although formula companies persuaded mothers in developing countries that bottle feeding is more modern and healthful than breastfeeding, the mothers typically did not have access to sanitary water to combine with the formula powder. Powdered infant formula goods are not sterilized and might be colonized with bacterial organisms.[58] Women in developing countries cannot afford expensive artificial formula to nourish their babies properly and cannot provide safe and clean containers for feeding.[27;137] Some cultural beliefs about breastfeeding might strongly influence the duration of exclusive breastfeeding and limit it to the early months; many mothers in developing nations might believe exclusive breastfeeding cannot satisfy their baby's nutritional needs and, therefore, introduce artificial formula feeds.[168]

Children who are formula fed are more likely to be exposed to potentially contaminated formula milk because of a lack of clean water and the presence of organisms such as *Enterobacter sakazakii* in powdered milk.[18] Multiple researchers have demonstrated an association between bacterial colonization of dried formula and infection among infants fed with the products.[58] Salmonella and other constituents of the Enterobacteriaceae family have been found in the majority of the reported cases in one study.[58]

Enterobacter sakazakii is an infective organism that has been found in artificial baby milk powdered formula and other foods in another study.[28] This organism is characterized as a Gram-negative, rod-shape bacterium that can cause invasive infection with high death rates in newborns.[57] *Enterobacter sakazakii* has an increased resistance to heat, which might play a vital role in its ability to colonize in powdered formula.[58] According to Bowen and Braden,[28] *Enterobacter sakazakii* kills 40 to 80 percent of all infected infants. Drudy, Mullane, Quinn, Wall, and Fanning reported,[52] "This bacterium is an emerging opportunistic pathogen that is associated with rare but life-threatening cases of meningitis, necrotizing enterocolitis, and sepsis in premature and full-term infants" (p. 996). The hazard is great because powered milk is not sterile and provides a good medium for bacterial growth because of prolonged periods of storage and administration at room temperature.[57]

The contagion is alarming because clinicians might not be aware of the potential risk for infection when administering non-sterile powered formula. Formula feeding might be routine in the healthcare setting, despite scientific evidence that formula could be and has been contaminated with infective organisms. Mothers might be discouraged from breastfeeding their babies because of concerns regarding toxins in their own milk, without considering the toxins that might be in the powdered formula.

Infants exposed to formula-feeding are more likely than their exclusively breastfed peers to suffer from acute illnesses, such as diarrhea, ear infections, pneumonia, meningitis,[156] and acute respiratory infections.[107] Formula-fed infants are also more likely to suffer from chronic illnesses and conditions such as sudden infant death syndrome (SIDS), obesity, childhood leukemia, asthma, and lowered IQ.[156] Since the

1900s, physicians have known "formula and the con-comitant dearth of human milk in an infant's diet can herald ill health for years"[156].

Studies have demonstrated "not only initiation of breastfeeding, but exclusivity and duration of breast-feeding, matter"[156](p. 6). A dose-response relation-ship exists between human health and breast-milk ingestion.[151] Babies who breastfeed for fewer than four weeks are five times more likely to die of SIDS than babies who breastfeed for more than sixteen weeks.[156] According to one study, the incidence of childhood obesity increases with the early introduction of for-mula-feeding.[126] Infants who breastfeed six months or less are approximately three times more likely to suf-fer from a malignancy than babies who breastfeed lon-ger than six months.[156] Lack of knowledge and proper support sustain the belief that artificial baby milk and breast milk are equivalent.[126]

Opposing Views to Breastfeeding

A large number of health workers and the public believe feeding artificial formula milk is the same as breastfeeding.[148] Mothers who choose to feed their in-fants by giving them artificial formula do so for many reasons. One reason might be the lack of knowledge of the benefits of breast milk. Other reasons might include previous problems with breastfeeding, per-ceived low milk supply, anxiety, and health issues.[44] A mother might also need to work and leave the baby with the father or a caretaker for several hours at a time.[150] Some mothers choose to formula feed their infants based on health-worker recommendations and the influence of corporate advertising.[126] Despite the fact that formula is not able to provide the multiple layers of disease protection that breast milk can, formula does fulfill the role of maintaining growth and development within normal limits.[148]

Artificially feeding an infant might give a mother the freedom of not having to be the only family member able to feed the infant. Formula feeding might provide convenience and flexibility in a working mother's life and help her know that her infant is being fed while she is away.[77] A formula-feeding mother depends on time to determine her child's meals and frequency of feeds rather than on the demand of the child to be fed, which provides a sense of flexibility and convenience.[77]

Artificial feeding might be necessary if a child is abandoned or orphaned or if a mother's health does not permit her to breastfeed. A mother might be too ill with cancer and be receiving chemotherapy, which is a contraindication for breastfeeding. According to Fulton and Moore,[73] breastfeeding is not recommended for infants of mothers who are undergoing long-term chemotherapy. Breastfeeding should be halted for a time determined by the type of medication used. Not all medications are contraindicated during breastfeeding. Some contraindicated drugs include bromocriptine, cyclophosphamide, cyclosporine, doxorubicin, ergotamine, lithium, methotrexate, and phencyclidine.[77]

Other contraindications or needs for supplementation to breastfeeding include insufficient maternal breast tissue as a result of breast reduction surgery, which might reduce the amount of milk produced.[38] If a mother has a habit of drug abuse, has a communicable disease such as active tuberculosis,[150] or is positive for HIV,[126;150] international agencies such as UNAIDS, UNICEF, and the WHO do not recommend breastfeeding.[109] Taha et al. reported breastfeeding is the most significant route of postnatal HIV transmission from mother to infant.[137] Mother-to-child transmission of HIV can happen any time during pregnancy, labor and delivery, or breastfeeding. Feeding a child directly from the breast is responsible for 90 percent of HIV global infections in children.[109;149] In breastfed infants, up to one-third of the total HIV transmission rate occurred after birth.[149;109] According to Orne-Gliemann et al.,[110] "Exclusive breastfeeding was identified as a mother-to-child transmission risk factor by 27.1 percent in 2002 and by 55.8 percent of respondents in 2004" when evaluating the influence of a prevention campaign on mother-to-child transmission of HIV in Zimbabwe. Piwoz and Ross contended,[116] "WHO recommends avoidance of all BF [breastfeeding] when replacement feeding (RF) is affordable, feasible, acceptable, sustainable, and safe" (p. 1113). Weinberg posited if continuous access to nutritionally sufficient breast-milk substitutes can be provided and safely prepared, HIV-infected women should be advised against breastfeeding their infants.

The fundamental supposition is that breastfeeding is rarely contraindicated during maternal infection, but microorganisms were found in colostrum and breast milk.[92] Few organisms were transmitted through breast milk to cause the infant clinically significant infections; the organisms that were transmitted included the HIV1 and human T-lymphotrophic virus I. Other organisms, such as group B streptococci, rarely caused infection when transmitted by breast milk. Weighing the benefits of breastfeeding against the potential risk for transmission is a dilemma that mothers face in making the decision about probable infection of an infant or child through breast milk.[92] Regardless of the dilemma in the decision-making process of mothers infected with HIV regarding feeding their infants, replacement feeding is recommended when it is "affordable, feasible, acceptable, sustainable, and safe."[21]

Current Health Findings in Saudi Arabia

A study conducted on the prevalence of obesity and inactivity in Saudi Arabia determined a need exists to institute programs to promote awareness among the population of the health hazards and means of control of obesity.[3;7] Health professionals define obesity as a BMI ≥ 30 kg/m^2,[59] and the definition of overweight is a BMI of 25.0–29.9 kg/m^2.[102] The evidence of a high prevalence of overweight and obesity among Saudi individuals is overwhelming, with Saudi females having the highest frequency of obesity.[7] Al Nozha, Al-Hazzaa, et al. proposed that because the natural occurrence of obesity increases with age, and considering that the majority of the Saudi population is currently less than thirty years old, the scale of obesity might be even greater in the coming years.[7] Further findings indicated a high prevalence of childhood obesity and recommended early health education programs on the appropriate choice of diet for growth, health, and longevity.[3]

Research demonstrated the number of patients with diabetes mellitus in Saudi Arabia has increased drastically. Diabetes is an epidemic in Saudi Arabia.[1] Al AlSheikh noted, "Almost one Saudi in four beyond the age of 30 has diabetes mellitus costing the government $800 per month" (para. 6). This high incidence of diabetes is because most of the population does not understand the disease and its consequences.[1] Poor diabetic control leads to many complications that require hospitalization and sometimes severe and drastic measures to help keep the patient alive; some individuals do not understand diabetes is preventable and can be managed once diagnosed.[1] Diabetes is a chronic burdensome disease, and it might be of interest to Saudi Arabians to combine efforts to reduce the potential numbers of diabetic patients.

Evidence from research indicated obesity, a sedentary lifestyle, and a lack of breastfeeding are precursors to type-2 diabetes. Al Nuaim reported age, obesity, and family history of diabetes mellitus were associated with having diabetes in Saudi Arabia.[8] The characteristics are considered normal in Saudi Arabia because of their high prevalence, although they are easily prevented and reversed. Al Nuaim stressed the need to build a multidisciplinary approach for the Saudi population, giving special attention to prevention of the disease. Al Nuaim contended, "Considering the young nature of [the] Saudi population, the prevalence is expected to increase in the near future" (p. 602). Attitudes must change, especially attitudes that consider the presence of an acute medical condition more important than glycemic control and let it overshadow the significance of glycemic control. Although diabetes might be considered a harmless companion unworthy of care and attention, the medical community is aware that diabetes is harmful and can lead to serious medical complications.

With the high prevalence of obesity and diabetes in Saudi Arabia, it is easy to understand the high prevalence of hypertension. A study conducted in 1998 on the prevalence of hypertension in Saudi Arabia indicated in a sample of 14,660 adult Saudis (males = 6,162; females = 8,498) the identified prevalence ranged from 1.4 to 18.71 percent in males and from 0.9 to 14 percent in females.[56] If the community was educated on the importance of breastfeeding and its role in reducing risk for developing hypertension in later stages in life, families might be more likely to participate in the national effort to lower health expenditures and increase the health status of the population as a whole.

Evidence also indicates that the overall health status of the Saudi population seems to be declining and the incidence of carcinomas is increasing. A study conducted in 2001 to evaluate the outline and pattern of male and female breast disease in 953 Saudi Arabians, with a mean age of forty-nine years reported 31.5 percent of all lesions were malignant.[93] Ductal carcinoma of the breast was the most common (80%), followed by lobular carcinoma of the breast (5.5%). Jamal's study confirmed the numbers with similar results.[83] In a study on the pattern of breast disease in a teaching hospital in the city of Jeddah, Jamal reported malignant lesions appeared in 32.5 percent of patients, with a mean patient age of 48.49 years. The malignancies most commonly reported were ductal carcinoma (88%) and lobular carcinoma (4.5%). Mansoor, Zahrani, and Abdul

Aziz contended,[94] "Colorectal carcinoma showed frequent presentation in our population" (p. 322).

Carcinomas have a strong presence in Saudi Arabia, prompting the establishment of the National Cancer Registry in Saudi Arabia in 1992.[10] Since January 1994, all cancer cases of Saudi and non-Saudi residents in Saudi Arabia have been registered with the National Cancer Registry. Results indicated 66 percent of 1,833 reported cases of primary gastrointestinal malignancies were Saudi Arabian.[10]

Patterns of Breastfeeding in Saudi Arabia

A pattern of decline exists in the exclusive breastfeeding practices of Saudi women. Partial breastfeeding is the dominant practice, and exclusive breastfeeding is very rare.[108] Partial breastfeeding rates in the western region of Saudi Arabia reached 90 percent for infants in the first six months of life, but dropped to 72 percent after the first six months.[60] Al-Othman et al. noted,[9] "Approximately 73% of the mothers breastfed their children initially but only 37.6% are currently [after 6 months] breastfeeding their children" (p. 909). Shawky and Abalkhahil noted in their study that breastfeeding declined quickly within the first year of a child's life in Saudi Arabia.[129] The most common reason for the early introduction of bottle-feeding cited by Al-Jassir et al. was that mothers perceived breast milk as inadequate. The reasons given by Fida and Al-Aama in their research samples for switching from breastfeeding to formula feeding were inadequate milk supply (50%), working mothers (12.7%), and lifestyle (10%).

Although inadequate milk supply, working mothers, and lifestyle are common reasons for the early introduction of bottle-feeding, a gap exists in the literature that does not address why these are the reasons in Saudi Arabia. Bystrova et al.'s study on early lactation concluded complex factors might influence or regulate milk production.[35] The results of the study indicated hospital ward routines influenced milk production and indicated a need for further research. Many factors, some internal and some external, might persuade a mother to discontinue breastfeeding. Internal factors might include self-esteem, perceptions about milk supply, and the need to work. External factors not mentioned in recent studies include socioeconomic status, education levels, health specialist advice, hospital ward practices, and marketing and advertising of formula manufacturing companies.

Proper breastfeeding practice should be promoted as early as the antenatal period.[129] Al-Jassir et al. posited, "There is a need to revise the media campaign for promoting breastfeeding utilizing the instructions and guidance from the Holy Quran and Hadiths" (p. 1). An Islamic country must practice not only the teachings of its governing religion, but also the scientifically proven standard for infant feeding to combat health concerns for the nation such as obesity, diabetes, hypertension, and cancer. Wright et al. wrote,[167] "Increasing the proportion of exclusively breastfed infants seems to be an effective means of reducing infant illness at the community level" (para. 5). A reduction in morbidity and mortality is associated with breastfeeding and is of significant magnitude to be of public health significance.[84]

One of the major problems with breastfeeding sustenance and infant feeding is the misconception mothers have about adequacy of milk supply and feeding patterns. In a study of Saudi women, Al-Othman et al. reported approximately 73 percent of the mothers breastfed their children initially, but only 37.6 percent continued to do so after approximately six months. The majority of mothers initiated breastfeeding one to eight hours after delivery, and 63 percent added supplementary foods to their children's diets at four to eight months of age. According to Fida and Al-Aama, the most frequent difficulty reported in maintaining breastfeeding among Saudi women was a mistaken belief concerning the adequacy of their milk supply. Little is known about women's perceptions regarding the need for prenatal education and preparation for motherhood. A detailed understanding of the central phenomenon and its complexities is needed to increase the numbers of mothers who exclusively breastfeed their infants.

Current Research

Common reasons for the early introduction of bottle-feeding are inadequate breast-milk supply, being a working mother, and lifestyle.[5;60] However, the literature did not address why these are the common reasons in Saudi Arabia. My dissertation study was an empirical phenomenological study that involved exploring an area of research that filled a void in the existing literature. A need existed to gain deeper understanding of issues pertaining to the specific problem of the partial breastfeeding patterns of Saudi women.

Prior to the study, limited information was available on the reasons behind Saudi mothers' lactation patterns and breastfeeding decisions. Hoping to close the gap in the literature, I chose to interview mothers and learn from them in an effort to increase peer-reviewed research that explains why partial breastfeeding is the most common method of infant feeding and whether exclusive breastfeeding exists at all in Saudi Arabia. The ultimate goal was to improve breastfeeding rates for the improvement of health status in the Kingdom. This book and the research that it is based on might help future health professionals establish stronger initiation programs for breastfeeding to protect people from diseases such as obesity, diabetes, hypertension, and cancer.

Health findings in Saudi Arabia indicate the high prevalence of obesity, which drives the need to institute programs for the promotion and increased awareness among the Saudi population of the health hazards of diabetes and the means of controlling this disease.[3] The evidence of a high prevalence of overweight and obesity among Saudi individuals is overwhelming.[11] Furthermore, the patterns of exclusive breastfeeding in Saudi Arabia are declining, which might be a reason for the increased obesity numbers seen in the population. Partial breastfeeding with artificial formula milk is the dominant practice, and exclusive breastfeeding is rare.[108] One of the major problems with breastfeeding sustenance and infant feeding is the misconception mothers have about the adequacy of their milk supply and the belief that breastmilk and artificial formula milk are equal, despite the fact that artificial milk might cause babies to be obese.

The aim of international organizations such as UNICEF and the WHO is to create a global environment in which women are empowered to begin skin-to-skin contact with their infants and initiate breastfeeding immediately after birth, to exclusively breastfeed for the first six months, and to maintain breastfeeding for two years or more with age-appropriate, responsive, and complementary feeding with regular table food. In an effort to make the goal of UNICEF attainable, the current involved an attempt to reinforce the breastfeeding culture in the Saudi community and defend against a bottle-feeding culture by providing evidence that might sway women in the direction of exclusive breastfeeding.

The purpose of my dissertation study was to generate descriptions for a better understanding of lactation patterns, to explore perceptions about prenatal education and preparation for motherhood, and to gain further understanding of the reasons that underlie Saudi women's lack of exclusive breastfeeding after delivery. The main objective was to discover and configure meaning that would lead to a deeper understanding of the influences on Saudi women's decisions in Jeddah regarding whether or not to breastfeed. The information that came out of the study could be used to improve a mother's understanding of breastfeeding or be used to design prenatal education classes that might enhance a woman's experience as a mother and ultimately help them make decisions in their infant's best interest. It is hoped that this study contributes knowledge that might help researchers to understand the nature of the problem, for intervention purposes, that improves breastfeeding rates in Saudi Arabia and to allows health-care leaders to encourage necessary changes to enable and promote breastfeeding.

Mothers were interviewed with open-ended questions that allowed them to express their perceptions freely about prenatal education and the concept of preparation for motherhood. This allowed the mothers to share their own stories to generate common factors and allowed investigation of their responses for external influences on the decisions made by the Saudi mothers. The intentional selection of individuals from a relevant group allowed for the learning, understanding, and in-depth exploration of this central social phenomenon.[47] The sample consisted of twenty Saudi women between the ages of twenty-one and thirty-five years who resided in Jeddah, a western province of Saudi Arabia, with infants aged newborn to four months. This style of qualitative research is useful when the intention is to learn how people manage their lives in the context of existing or potential health matters and their resulting decisions.[53]

Findings

The research question was designed to investigate the influences that caused mothers in Saudi Arabia to partially breastfeed their infants. The research question had two sub-questions. The first sub-question aimed to investigate the influences that affect a mother's feeding decisions. The second sub-question aimed to investigate the influences that affect a mother's decision to adopt partial breastfeeding.

Qualitative research usually involves open-ended and general research questions that allow the flow of information to be expressed to create categories of concepts.[127] The main categories that emerged from within the data were as follows: (a) experiences that made breastfeeding difficult, (b) influences that inclined mothers to breastfeed at all, and (c) influences that inclined mothers to use breastfeeding alternatives.

Experiences that made breastfeeding difficult was first of the three main categories that emerged through the analysis process. The following elements comprised this category: (a) breastfeeding is accepted but not supported, (b) the lack of breastfeeding education techniques, (c) guests and visitors around, (d) pressure from older female family members, (e) public places and venues, (f) self-esteem and body image, (g) hospital discouragement, (h) criticism of how the mother takes care of her baby, (i) husbands being passive, and (j) having other children to take care of.

The following are examples of the statements made by the mothers. The element *breastfeeding is accepted but not supported* refers to a mother's outlook on society's opinion of breastfeeding: "[Breastfeeding is] accepted but it is not supported…. The moment you face any problems, the easiest thing for them to say is, 'C'mon just give him a bottle, or just stop breastfeeding.'" The element *lack of breastfeeding education techniques* refers to a mother's inexperience in positioning a baby to latch on to breastfeed: "When they got me my baby to the room for the first time, the first problem I faced was not having control on the baby's position [I didn't know how to hold him]." The element *guests and visitors around* refers to a mother's lack of privacy and discomfort with having family and friends around the hospital and the home immediately after delivering a baby and trying to breastfeed: "When we first deliver, it's hard to receive visitors and bond with your baby." The element *pressure from older female family members* refers to mothers, grandmothers, and aunts imposing their unsolicited opinions, advice, and techniques onto a mother with respect to breastfeeding: "They keep telling me: you don't have milk! And you have small breasts you won't get any milk! It made me upset." The element *public places and venues* refers to a mother's discomfort in being in public while breastfeeding or the avoidance of going in public by a mother because of breastfeeding: "I can't feed in public because there are no places for breastfeeding." The element *self-esteem and body image* refers to a mother's dissatisfaction with the physical appearances of her breasts and body due to the effects of pregnancy and breastfeeding: "Of course it takes time to get used to your body image, the stretch marks and all that." The element *hospital discouragement* refers to the practice of hospital staff discouraging breastfeeding after delivery because of the convenience of breastfeeding alternatives: "The only people who didn't support me were nurses in the hospital." The element *criticism of how a mother takes care of her baby* refers to the negative feedback a mother receives from others with respect to her breastfeeding practices: "Everyone sits and stares at you like you are a bad mother and you don't know what you're doing." The element *husbands being passive* refers to the instances where a mother's husband is removed from the decisions regarding breastfeeding: "[My husband] supports everything I say. He's never against me, but he never acts, he is always passive." Last, the element *having to take care of other children* refers to the difficulty a mother experiences in having to tend to other children while trying to breastfeed: "Then you end up staying up late and of course [you] can't wake up to give your children their breakfast or take them to school."

One important item to note is that the main category, *experiences that made breastfeeding difficult,* only included the difficulties mothers faced in choosing to exclusively breastfeed. The elements of that main category referred to instances when a mother was influenced by external factors to make a choice to include breastmilk alternatives in her lactation patterns. The next two main categories, *influences that inclined mothers to breastfeed at all* and *influences that inclined mothers to use breastfeeding alternatives* addressed this issue even more specifically.

The second main category derived from the phenomenological reduction process was the *influences that inclined a mother to choose to breastfeed at all.* The following elements made up this category: (a) breastfeeding was always the mother's choice, (b) husband is supportive of breastfeeding, (c) importance of the mother-child bond, (d) family support from females, (e) physician or healthcare advice, (f) breastfeeding helps with immunity and health, (g) friend's support, (h) educational support to breastfeed, and (i) faith or religious support.

Here are examples of statements made by the mothers interviewed. The element *breastfeeding was always the mother's choice* refers to the intangible influence on a mother's attitude that she did not want to employ an alternative to breastfeeding: "I wanted to breastfeed from the beginning." The element *husband is supportive of breastfeeding* refers to a mother's husband playing a positive and active role in the choice to breastfeed: "My husband really wishes that I only breastfeed." The element *importance of the mother-child bond* refers to the importance a mother places on the bond that develops between her and her child during the breastfeeding process: "The first couple of days are very important to establish the bond between the mother and the baby." The element *family support from females* refers to older female family members who are supportive of breastfeeding: "I heard about the center from family, my grandmother." The element *physician or health-care advice* refers to the advice a mother receives from her doctor or other health-care professionals that encourages breastfeeding: "My physician told me about Al Bidayah center when I was pregnant with my first daughter. He knew I was BF and directed me to your center for support and information." The element *breastfeeding helps with immunity and health* refers to the benefits a child receives from breastfeeding in terms of antibodies and proper amounts of vitamins and proteins: "It gives immunity to the baby more than the formula," "He might have immunity from the milk but still it's also about good nutrition." The element *friend's support* refers to a mother's friends encouraging the use of breastfeeding: "I remember I heard a friend talking about the importance of breastfeeding." The element *receiving educational support to breastfeed* refers to an educational experience a mother encounters that leads her to choose breastfeeding: "The information I got from the lactation control center [and the staff's] availability and help" and "I always knew that breastfeeding is important; I had little previous information about it from friends who have been breastfeeding." Last, the element *faith or religious support* refers to the religious and spiritual guidance and support a mother experiences in choosing to breastfeed: "The only thing that helped me continue was God's help and after that the support I had from some friends."

The findings from the second main category, *influences that led a mother to choose to breastfeed*, revealed that the participants reported they were influenced to breastfeed because they always had breastfeeding as the only option in mind, their husbands were supportive of them choosing to breastfeed, and they placed importance on the bond between mother and child developed through breastfeeding. Many of the mothers reported they were influenced to breastfeed because of the support they received from their friends and advice they received from their doctors and other healthcare professionals. Some of the mothers stated the antibodies and health benefits influenced their decision to breastfeed, and others stated that education on breastfeeding and spiritual or religious support were reasons for choosing to breastfeeding.

The third main category derived from the phenomenological reduction processes was the *influences that led a mother to use alternatives to breastfeeding*. The following elements were identified in the reduction process for the third main category: (a) to relieve the pressure from family members, (b) formula was convenient, (c) mother felt she did not have enough milk, (d) wanted child to sleep at night, (e) wanted to socialize, (f) wanted child to gain weight, and (g) health problems for the mother.

Here are examples of statements made by the mothers I interviewed. The element *to relieve the pressure from family members* refers to the instances when a mother uses formula due to the advice of assertive family members (especially female relatives) recommending alternatives to breastfeeding: "I felt like everyone wanted to take control and everyone was judging my decision like water for example—'Why don't you give him water? We give all our kids water. What's wrong with water?' I knew I shouldn't give him water, I just didn't know how to defend it. Pressure everywhere! They tell me, 'He is losing weight. Why are you ignoring it? You're being stubborn.' And now if you ask me when I started introducing formula…I decided by myself after all the pressure when he started losing weight. I thought maybe that would relieve me from the pressure."

This element also refers to the case where older female family members want to re-experience their own motherhood by being able to feed an infant themselves with a bottle of artificial formula: "Even the bottle [can] create a bond between mother [or person who feeds] and baby and that's what [some] mothers want. BF time makes it exclusive for the mom." The element *formula was convenient* refers to the extra time and effort bypassed when using an alternative to breastfeeding: "I feel that it is easier to just give formula. Maybe it is irresponsible; I should express, but it is very hard to express. But I feel that it is exhausting, and my mother tells me to make him used to the artificial milk." The element *mother felt she did not have enough milk* refers to a mother using formula because she feels her milk production is low: "Sometimes I give him an external formula feed because I have no milk. I give him time and try, but I am forced to give him formula because I don't have enough milk." The element *wanted child to sleep at night* refers to the instances where a mother wants her baby to sleep longer during the night, so she gives the baby a bottle of artificial formula: "She would sleep through the night when she had formula," "Before I go to sleep I give him a bottle of formula, just so he can sleep well and I can sleep." The element *wanted to socialize* refers to the convenience for a mother of not being embarrassed to breastfeed at social gatherings: "Every time I need to feed my baby I need to leave the room. Especially in family gatherings, I feed him formula. I always feed him formula when we are out, but as soon as I leave the house I feed formulas." The element *wanted child to gain weight* refers to a mother using artificial formula because she thinks her baby is not getting sufficient nutrition: "I started giving formula at night so he sleeps well and to relieve pressure I also want him to gain weight." The element *health problems for the mother* refers to instances in the hospital immediately after delivery where a mother doesn't want to risk her health by breastfeeding: "I didn't have the knowledge and I didn't want to jeopardize my baby's health so of course I gave him [formula]."

Many of the participants reported they chose breastfeeding alternatives to relieve the influencing pressure from older female family members. Many of the mothers also reported using alternatives because it was convenient with respect to time and effort and addressed the issue of possibly not having enough milk. Some mothers used alternatives because they believed it would help their child sleep better at night, and other mothers stated that they used alternatives because they wanted to go out in public, wanted their child to gain weight, or did not want to risk their own health or the health of their baby by breastfeeding.

The development of categories and structure of meaning allowed the reflection and construction of concepts that related the subjective experiences to cognitive social learning theories. The connection and construction of relationships allowed further understanding and a possible explanation of the phenomenon of partial breastfeeding in Saudi Arabia. The explanation is that local feeding practices are a social practice that one mother models and might impose on another. Researcher interpretations centered on the notion that female elders influence Saudi women's infant feeding practices. Additional findings included the importance of prenatal education for the mother and her family, the need for emotional support of the breastfeeding mother, and improved physician and hospital practices regarding breastfeeding promotion, protection, and support.

Interpretations

The guiding research question was designed to investigate the social influences that cause mothers in Saudi Arabia to choose partial breastfeeding to nourish their infants. The research sub-questions aimed to investigate the experiences that lead a mother to make decisions regarding feeding methods and guide her to practice partial breastfeeding. In the study, three main categories emerged: (a) experiences that made breastfeeding difficult, (b) influences that led mothers to breastfeed at all, and (c) influences that led mothers to use breastfeeding alternatives.

The majority of the mothers reported experiencing difficulty in trying to breastfeed because society is not supportive. The mothers also described a lack of breastfeeding education techniques as a big problem. Guests and visitors in the mother's hospital room caused difficulty for the participants. Pressure from older female family members and time spent in public places each elicited a strong response from the participants as major reasons for not being able to practice exclusive breastfeeding. These findings are consistent with the findings of Betzold et al.,[24] who noted the beliefs and values of other women, their families, the workplace, and health professionals involved in their care, as well as formula milk advertisements, can strongly direct the decision to breastfeed or not to breastfeed. Earlier research indicated the norms and beliefs must be positively influenced and directed toward proper infant-feeding practices that support, promote, and protect breastfeeding practices.[24]

The participants mentioned influences that inclined them to breastfeed at all as being preexisting attitudes: breastfeeding was always their preference, their husbands were supportive of breastfeeding, and breastfeeding was important to a mother-child bond. The participating mothers also mentioned that female friends' and family members' support and physicians' or healthcare providers' advice were positive influences on their lactation practices. Many of the mothers reported in depth that their knowledge and understanding of the health and immunological benefits of breastfeeding motivated them to include breastfeeding in their infant feeding practices.

Two elements emerged equally as being a strong influence for mothers' decisions to use breastfeeding alternatives: to relieve the pressure from family members and the formula was convenient. Many mothers said they did not feel they had enough breast milk to breastfeed their child exclusively. Some of the participants gave formula to their children at night because they wanted them sleep well. Other mothers reported that their lifestyles of frequent social gatherings did not allow them to breastfeed comfortably; this was one of the main influences that inclined them to use breastfeeding alternatives. A few of the mothers said they wanted their children to gain weight so they gave artificial formula to *nourish them well.* Not many mothers reported having health problems that prohibited the process of breastfeeding.

A mother is more inclined to use artificial feeding methods than breastfeeding because of social and environmental pressures that she cannot withstand, personal feelings of convenience, misinformation about infant nutrition, and misinformation about breastfeeding and breast milk supply. The three main categories that emerged from elements reported by the participants are greatly personal, social, and environmental, which highlights that a mother's lactation patterns and infant feeding decisions are based on her environment. The lack of exclusive breastfeeding in Saudi Arabia is due to the social environment's attitude shift toward and in favor of artificial formula feeding and only partial breastfeeding.

The following passage contains segments of the combined interview transcripts from the three interviews with Participant 1. The passage is an example that illustrates the subjective concepts that emerged during the data collection process. From these concepts, the data were reduced into categories as discussed above.

Researcher: How did you become a client at Al Bidayah Breastfeeding Resource and Women's Awareness Center and what do you personally know about breastfeeding?

Participant 1: I wanted to breastfeed from the beginning. I didn't have much information about breastfeeding, but it felt like the right thing to do. The center offered awareness classes about breastfeeding so I decided to join. I always knew that breastfeeding is important; I had little previous information about it from friends who have been breastfeeding. People never say that breastfeeding is difficult. They keep telling me, "You don't have milk!" and "You have small breasts, you won't get any milk!" It made me upset. There is no such thing as no milk.

Researcher: What do you think about the whole idea of breastfeeding in general?

Participant 1: I always had this image of a mother nursing her child from older women around me. It never occurred to me that breastfeeding was that important for the baby. I didn't know it was that different from the formula. I mean, I knew that breastfeeding is better but just because it was natural and contained antibodies. After I heard from my friends what they've learned from the course and seen them apply it, I could see the bond and intimacy between them and their babies. I don't think it's a very good idea to breastfeed in public because that way you lose the intimacy that you share with your baby.

Researcher: How did your perception change after you started breastfeeding?

Participant 1: After I gave birth, I made sure that I started breastfeeding immediately and for me that was a great experience! I was able to breastfeed even though my baby had a small problem and I almost lost hope. When I was finally able to breastfeed, it felt like the right beginning. When they got me my baby to the room for the first time, the first problem I faced was not having control on the baby's position; I didn't know how to handle him. Instead of concentrating on how the baby is latched on, I spent the whole time focusing on my hands and trying to support the baby. I had about six pillows with me at the hospital, yet I was still not relaxed.

Researcher: In our society is breastfeeding accepted or not?

Participant 1: Yes, it is accepted, but it is not supported.

Researcher: Elaborate please.

Participant 1: Well everyone around you tells you [that] you should breastfeed—your mother, relatives, and even friends who never did breastfeed, but the moment you face any problems, the easiest thing for them to say is, "C'mon just give him a bottle," or "Just stop breastfeeding." They don't even want to hear what you have to say about the new research about its importance. It is like [they are] saying if it's difficult then just stop breastfeeding.

Who Cares?

The results of this research helped determine the factors that influence Saudi Arabian women in Jeddah not to exclusively breastfeed their infants. The results can be applied in practice in a variety of ways. The study results can improve a woman's understanding of the situation that she may face or provide information to design prenatal education classes that might enhance women's experiences as mothers to help them make decisions in their infants' best interests. The findings might assist in creating a focus for the design of a national breastfeeding campaign in Saudi Arabia and other similar programs that could use the results as theoretical support.

The study indicated that personal beliefs and knowledge, social models and support, and environmental trends heavily influence Saudi mothers' lactation patterns and infant feeding decisions. The descriptions of experiences might be of significance based on the information available to help health-care leaders encourage necessary changes in hospital practices, business practices involved in baby food marketing, maternity laws, and cultural norms to enable and promote breastfeeding. The configured meaning might also be of significance to assist in providing evidence for a need for prenatal breastfeeding education and to offer data that might support the revision of certain maternity protection laws and the creation of mother- and baby-friendly workplaces. The evidence that has emerged gives rise to the concern that if these elements are not addressed, Saudi women will continue current infant feeding practices and will not be able to exclusively breastfeed ever again. Therefore, the prevalence of breastfeeding in the region will not improve.

Although the current study was limited to Saudi Arabian women in the city of Jeddah, the results might carefully be applied elsewhere. If other groups of women describe the same influences as the Saudi Arabian influences, the study's results could have the same practical uses to these groups of women. The application of this study to other groups of women must be done carefully and not without further verification of reliability. Lastly, the findings could be the foundation for future studies and inspire the research of topics closely related to the topic of the study.

Conclusions

The quest to answer the research questions led to some conclusions regarding the influences that cause women to breastfeed or not to breastfeed their children. The most common experiences that made breastfeeding difficult were the findings that breastfeeding is accepted but not supported, the lack of breastfeeding education, having guests, pressure from older female family members, and being in public. Other than the lack of breastfeeding education, this investigation indicated that Saudi women are concerned with others' opinions in their environment regarding breastfeeding. The following are the most influential factors that lead a mother to choose to breastfeed: breastfeeding is their personal preference, support of female family members or husbands, and the importance of a mother-child bond. These elements are based on proper knowledge and understanding of the benefits of breastfeeding. The most influential factors that lead a mother to use breastfeeding alternatives are to relieve pressure from family members and convenience. Interestingly, neither of these most influential factors had any direct regard for the infant.

A mother is more prone to use artificial feeding methods rather than breastfeeding due to social and environmental pressures that she cannot endure, personal feelings of convenience, misinformation about infant nutrition, and misinformation about breastfeeding and breast-milk supply. The lack of exclusive breastfeeding in Saudi Arabia is a result of the social environment's attitude shift toward partial breastfeeding.

MY EXPERIENCE AND WHAT I HAVE LEARNED

❧

All mammals breastfeed their young, including whales and dolphins; this is what differentiates mammals from all other creatures. Mammary glands (breast tissue) play a very large role in the reproduction stages of the mammalian species. Humans are characterized as mammals because we have the ability to nurture and breastfeed our young. Many mammals show that *early* contact with their young soon after birth holds an important place in the protection of motherly behavior and breastfeeding. Breastfeeding is natural, biological, and mammalian.

Breastfeeding is the natural continuation of childbearing. It is the external nourishment and caring that an infant needs to continue to grow and develop. I have a strong belief regarding the importance of the initiation of breastfeeding within the first thirty minutes after normal delivery and as soon as possible after cesarean sections (C-sections). Unfortunately, due to unnatural hospital and cultural practices in countries such as Saudi Arabia, a healthy newborn human is most likely to be separated from his or her mother while waiting for the mother's milk to *come in.* During this waiting period, the baby is unnecessarily supplemented by artificial formula. It is likely harmful for breastfeeding and for bonding, which is important for the development of a healthy mother-baby relationship.

I believe that hospital and social practices must be changed to allow mothers to put babies to the breast as soon as they are able, whether the milk *comes in* or not. It is only natural to do so. During the first hour of life, a baby will latch on instinctively and breastfeed well. However, after that hour the instinct to breastfeed is lost, especially if the baby is given an artificial bottle to feed. With nature interrupted, the baby will become nipple confused and may reject the breast.

Breastfeeding is an art learned by observation from female to female and that is passed on from mother to daughter, aunt to niece, sister to sister, and friend to friend. Breastfeeding is a learned behavior where mimicking what another mother practices with her baby is the essence of its success or failure. Breastfeeding is similar to dancing the waltz, in that the steps of the partners must be in line with each other, and if one partner dances one step offbeat, then both partners will be offbeat. Breastfeeding is a learned *art* like painting, carpentry, and other arts that require learned skill sets and intuitive talent; it is a skill that has basic steps for success. The ABCs and 123s of breastfeeding, if perfected, ensure successful exclusive breastfeeding. The basics can be learned through mimicking or from an expert who can teach the steps with clear instruction and scientific support.

Synchronize your bodies

Mother and baby must be synchronized and kept in close physical contact, breast to mouth, so that the mother's body can react appropriately to the baby's physical and nutritional needs. The mother's ability to make milk depends largely on the baby's demand. To understand this concept well, one must understand the physical relationship between a breastfeeding mother and her baby.

When a neonate is born, all the nutrients that were delivered through the umbilical cord from the placenta are immediately diverted to the breast. Production is slow unless the mother initiates breastfeeding early (within thirty minutes to one hour after delivery) and lets her body know that the baby is alive. When the infant latches on to the breast properly, there is a negative pressure pulling on the breast tissue as a result of the baby's suckling creating a demand. This pressure pulls the blood volume through the breast and into the baby's mouth in the form of colostrum and, later on, mature milk. Like a filter, the breast tissue transforms blood into milk with the assistance of prolactin and oxytocin. These hormones are high in the mother's blood due to direct breast stimulation by the baby that sends messages to the pituitary gland in the mother's brain. As soon as the baby ingests the colostrum during the first few days and properly stimulates the breast's nerves, mature milk begins to flow, encouraging higher milk volumes to be produced. This relationship must be renewed for each feed, so that the mother's body continues to make the proper amounts of milk for the baby's biological needs.

Many Middle Eastern mothers practice giving a baby teas to ease *tummy aches* or one formula feed at night to *encourage* sleep. This practice can easily disrupt the synchronization and, therefore, disrupt the amounts of milk that the mother produces for her baby, which might cause a drop in her milk supply. For example, on a random day the baby might need to feed twelve feeds at the breast to be satisfied, but the mother only feeds eleven feeds directly from the breast and gives the baby one external feed (tea or formula). The demand that is made directly on the breast from the baby is only for eleven feeds, so over time the mother's body will absorb the extra twelfth feed and only produce eleven as demanded by the baby. Soon the baby will grow and need more milk, say thirteen feeds, but the mother's body will only be producing eleven; with the increased milk demand, the baby will cry and the mother will be forced to increase the external feeds to two feeds instead of one.

The concept of *supply and demand* is the essence of breastfeeding. The more the baby demands directly from the breast, the more the breast will produce. If the baby needs twelve feeds a day, the mother's breast will produce those feeds. As the baby needs more and more milk with growth the demand will increase. Sometimes a baby may feed continuously for several days; this is known as *cluster feeding* and it is very normal. This cluster feeding time will last from 3 to 7 days and it usually begins around three weeks old. If the mother addresses the infant's hunger demands her milk supply will increase and the infant's urge to continuously feed will subside. The most important thing is for a mother to understand that this is normal and if she gives in to her baby's breastfeeding needs cluster feeding will pass sooner.

Latching On

Direct contact between a mother and baby is essential for successful breastfeeding. Pumping the breast no matter how effectively can not replace the important skin to skin contact of direct breastfeeding. The baby must be latched on well to the breast and suckle effectively to cause direct stimulation of the nerves under the areola of the breast. As the baby suckles with its lips flanged outward against the mother's skin, the mother's nerves are stimulated to send messages to her brain, specifically the pituitary gland, and in response, the pituitary gland releases two hormones into her bloodstream. These are the breastfeeding hormones, prolactin and oxytocin, that work on the breast tissue. Prolactin causes a chemical change in the breast, turning blood into milk, and the oxytocin works on contracting the fine smooth muscles in the breast to squeeze and express the milk out of the breast tissue through the ducts toward the nipple.

The breast is an organ with an anatomy that looks like a sponge or lung. It is full of alveoli and ducts, and behaves like a filter. We all know that a filter can be used to transform one type of liquid into another. Simply stated, with the appropriate pressure from the baby's latch and suckling, the blood rich in prolactin and oxytocin rushes through the breast which in turn transforms the blood directly into milk. The alignment of the baby's body is also very important for proper suckling. If the baby's body is twisted, the baby will not be able to latch on well. The baby must be lying flat on his or her side facing the mother. The baby's face, neck, and tummy should be in one line against the mother's tummy (tummy to tummy).

The perfect latch-on is essential for breastfeeding success and perfect suckling. If you swipe your tongue along the roof of your mouth, you will find the hard plate that extends all the way into the soft palette. During breastfeeding that involves proper suckling, the baby must grasp the breast tissue, pulling the nipple all the way back into the soft palette. The nipple is a hard tissue that will crack and tear if the baby suckles with it against the hard palette. Thus, it is important that the baby takes the nipple all the way back against the soft palette. If the baby has a sensitive palette and is not used to something touching the soft palette, he or she will gag. The gag reflex is naturally very high in this area of the mouth, and a nipple confused baby who gags can cause the mother to believe incorrectly that her baby is disgusted by her milk or that the baby is sensing that there is not enough milk. When a baby is exposed to a bottle, the gag reflex is heightened, causing what is known as nipple confusion, where the infant begins to suck rather than suckle. When a baby bottle feeds, the teat only extends to the hard palette, leaving the soft palette untouched and increasing its sensitivity. In addition, the baby must use the tongue as a stopper against the artificial teat to control the flow to lessen the chance of choking. The baby controls the flow from the bottle by sucking to draw milk out, then stopping the milk with the tongue to swallow and breathe. Bottle feeding trains the baby to suck and not suckle, making it more difficult to breastfeed.

Nipple confusion at the early age of one week can easily be corrected with finger feeding or the Islamic practice known as *tahneek*. The process is simple and allows the infant to suckle on an adult small finger (with the nail against the tongue) long enough to reduce soft palette sensitivity and to learn how to extend the tongue far enough over the gum ridge of the lower jaw. Extension of the tongue is important because the baby needs to use its tongue to express the breast and stimulate the breast nerves at the same time. If the roof of the baby's mouth (soft and hard palette) is sensitive, the baby will not be able to perform this task. Finger feeding, or tahneek, forces the tongue forward and reduces the sensitivity of the soft palette almost instantly.

Abu Buradah reported from Abu Musa, who said, "I had a new-born baby; I took him to the Prophet Muhammad, upon him be peace and blessings, who called him Ibrahim. The Prophet (peace be upon him) chewed a date then he took it and rubbed the inside of the baby's mouth with 't." Many believe that the sugary substance of the date is what benefits the baby, and some say that it was the Prophet's blessed saliva. However, from my practice and experience (I don't chew a date or use any sugary substance), it is the fact that Prophet Mohammad encouraged the infant to properly suckle his finger to encourage breastfeeding. The benefit of tahneek is the rubbing of the infant's mouth; this rubbing reduces sensitivity and encourages proper *suckling*.

Is the baby getting enough?

The golden yellow sticky substance (colostrum) secreted during the first days after delivery is important because it coats the baby's digestive tract to protect it from any external contaminants that can be ingested. The baby is born with a stomach that is not flexible and can only hold 5 ml of milk on the first day; thus, the baby feeds frequently and for short periods of time. Many mothers might think they do not have enough milk and that the baby is not satisfied; however, the frequent feeding and short feeding bouts are very normal and must not be interrupted to avoid interrupting the natural process of producing mature milk. As the mature milk begins to come in, the baby's stomach begins to expand and stretch, allowing it to retain more milk and by the end of the first week, the baby can hold 7 to 10 ml in the stomach.

A very common question for a breastfeeding mother to ask herself is, "Am I feeding my baby enough?" This question can be easily answered if a mother watches and monitors her baby closely. Important signs to look for are satiety after each feed, number of urine-filled diapers, and the color of the baby's stool. When a baby is satisfied, he or she cannot feed anymore; he or she will gently drop off the breast and fall asleep. A well fed baby will produce six to eight urine-filled diapers, and a mustard yellow colored stool.

After the establishment of the mature milk supply (usually one week after delivery) each of the mother's breasts will produce full meals for each feed. A full meal (feed) at one breast will include foremilk and hindmilk. The foremilk is a watery like substance that satisfies a baby's thirst, and the hindmilk is thick and fatty, satisfying a baby's hunger. A mother can tell if her baby has had too much foremilk or enough hindmilk from the color of the stool. If the stool is green, it means the baby has had too much foremilk and is not breastfeeding long enough on one breast. The baby will be colicky and unsatisfied. If the baby's stool is dark mustard yellow in color with fatty seeds, it means that the baby has had enough hindmilk and has breastfed long enough on one breast to be properly nourished. The baby will be in good spirits and be calm and easier to deal with. I often recommend that a mother time how long a baby sleeps away from the breast to decide which breast to feed from next rather than timing the length of the breastfeeding session on the breast. For example, a mother feeds her baby from the right breast and the baby comes off by choice and sleeps. If the baby sleeps for less than an hour and requests to be fed again, the mother should feed from the same breast. However, if the baby sleeps for an hour or longer and then requests to feed, the mother should feed from the other breast. The length of sleep away from the breast indicates to the mother if a baby has had a full feed from the initial breast. The shorter the length of the sleep, the less hindmilk the baby might have ingested. The longer the length of sleep, the more hindmilk the baby might have ingested.

Night feeding plays a role in milk supply. Night feeding is important for the success of breastfeeding because prolactin is secreted during the night. In order for a mother to breastfeed exclusively for six months, she must have the appropriate amounts of milk for her growing baby. A mother must maintain her prolactin levels by breastfeeding at night. A mother living in nature would not look at the time; a mother living in nature would act upon instinct letting her body do what it does best, which is nurture her baby.

When discussing night feeding with my clients, I often think of mothers who lived centuries ago. I tell them to think about the women who lived in nature and did natural things; they had no time keeping devices, technology, electricity, or safe man-made structures to live in. A woman in the desert would have lived in a tent; during the day she might have left the baby in the tent (protected from the heat) to complete her outdoor daily chores, coming back to feed her baby every few hours. However, during the night the baby would have been kept safe cradled in the mother's arms and left to breastfeed uninterrupted. It is natural for a mother and baby to be in close physical contact during the dark hours of the night. It is natural for a mother to be busy during the day with work or other children, but it is not natural for her to leave her baby unattended during the night. Therefore, based on biology and natural human behavior, prolactin is secreted at night to ensure the appropriate amount of milk is made for the next day. If there is no demand on her breast during the night, the prolactin hormones will drop, causing less milk to be made for the next day, which will decrease gradually and dry up over a few months. This is merciful for the mother, because if the baby no longer exists for some reason, the milk will reduce with the lack of demand on the breast at night.

As noted earlier, breastfeeding is an art, with basic steps needed to make it complete. As with any art form, be it painting, masonry, or carpentry, one learns from an expert. These art forms and many others require a set of skills that must be perfected and precise for the art to be successful. Breastfeeding is not like conception, which is only a natural bodily function. It is the complex continuation of childbirth and a transition into childrearing. These stages in the childrearing years are gradual and overlap during the first two years of life.

Pumping

It is important to pump before a breastfeed and not after. It is easier to express a full breast and feed the baby an empty breast. A mother's body will react positively toward her hungry baby, even if she had just pumped and the breast will naturally produce more milk for the feed, whereas she will not have a positive maternal reaction toward the pump, which will make it more difficult to pump an empty breast.

Milk volume is higher in the daytime and milk density is higher in the evenings. Therefore, pumping in the evening will not produce large amounts of milk to store. If a mother needs to leave her baby and provide ample amounts of milk while she is gone, it is best for her to pump both breasts at the same time first thing in the morning before she feeds her baby.

Rooming-In

The practice of rooming-in of the baby with the mother in the hospital during the early postpartum period is very important to understand, specifically for Middle Eastern cultures. It is a well-established tradition to visit the new mother in her hospital room, but this practice has encouraged mothers to leave their newborn infants in the hospital nursery with the nurses. The cultural reasoning behind this is so that the baby is not exposed to potential sicknesses from the visitors, to protect the baby from the evil eye that might cause death or illness, and to allow the mother to rest and not worry about the care of her newborn infant in the early days. However, rooming-in is essential for the maintenance of infant immunity and the reduction of morbidity and mortality. When the mother and baby are kept together, bonding is improved and the mother can instinctually and naturally address her infant's needs without hesitation. When the mother and baby are kept together, the baby is most protected physically and physiologically because the mother's body has a mature immune system that will automatically react to any pathogen that might cause illness and excrete that immunity into her milk supply for the baby. Rooming-in improves milk supply and secures proper latching-on techniques because the baby is not exposed to unnecessary bottle feeding by the usually overworked nurses.

Adoptive Breastfeeding

The issue of adoption in Islam is controversial. From my understanding, it is not recommended by Islamic teachings to adopt a child and give him or her a different name from the one given by the biological parents or family. However, there are many children who are brought into this world with unknown parents for many reasons that make it quite difficult to attribute a child to a specific family. Under Islamic law, many children are brought into a family as foster children and given a random name. The children are reared and cared for as family members in childhood, but not given any rights of biological relations or inheritance as an adult. The absence of these rights maintains the privileges of potential marriage within the family and independence from the family in adulthood.

There is one exception to the rule, which is breastfeeding. Breastfeeding an infant or child under the age of two years can improve the child's adoptive situation because breastfeeding gives the child the rights of birth. The Holy Quran clearly states "Let another woman suckle (the child) on the (mother's) behalf" (65:6), and the Hadith by Aisha (blessing of Allah upon her) says, "Breastfeeding denies what is denied by birth." These statements support the notion that other than the birth mother, any lactating woman can be the milk mother of a child and give that child the same birth rights as her own. It is agreed that in order for her to accomplish this she must feed an infant three to five satisfying feeds. A satisfying feed is approximated at around 50 ml of expressed breast milk; as soon as she has completed these three to five feeds, she is considered a milk-mother and has rights to the child just as much as his biological mother. This means the child will be a child to her husband, a sibling to her children, and a relative to all extended family members.

Any woman can breastfeed, whether she has recently delivered a baby or not. It is biologically possible for a woman to lactate or relactate, regardless of her childbearing status. I have experienced this possibility with two adoptive mothers. Both mothers were women who had been married for many years and had never conceived a child. Both mothers adopted and breastfed infants around the age of four months old with 250 ml of expressed breast milk under my supervision.

Lactation and milk expression took approximately two weeks. To encourage lactation, the mothers began by orally taking 60 mg of Domperidone a day and several cups of brewed Fenugreek while pumping and stimulating their breasts every two hours. During the first week, small beads of milk could be seen coming out of the breast; by the end of two weeks, the mothers were able to express 250 ml of breast milk, fulfilling the need for the five feeds to make the children their own. In both instances, as soon as the child was fed the full 250 ml, the mother ceased the medication and stopped pumping as the milk diminished naturally.

Adoptive breastfeeding is a beautiful option for couples who want a child and for a child who needs loving parents. Adoptive breastfeeding is a tool that can be used to improve lives. It forces the biological relationship to be primary to rearing an adopted infant. Through breastfeeding, nature has given women a means to give life, improve circumstances, and correct social problems.

Questions I Often Ask

If I gave you the choice to eat an *artificial* apple or a natural apple, which would you choose? I suppose you would choose the natural one, because the artificial one is made of an assortment of chemicals, preservatives, and sugar. So, why would you give your newborn child *artificial* milk? It is made of an assortment of chemicals, preservatives, sugar, and adjusted cow milk or soymilk proteins.

How would we feed our infants if for some reason the world faced an economic crisis that shut down all artificial milk factories? How would women know how to breastfeed if we don't keep the art of breastfeeding alive? How would our daughters learn how to breastfeed if we don't role model for them? Do we have to wait for war, death, and disease before we realize the value of keeping our babies perfectly nourished and healthy?

∾✵∾

Breastfeeding and Ramadan

Many women wonder if they should fast while they're breastfeeding, and some women choose not to breastfeed so that they can fast during Ramadan. The good news is that a mother probably doesn't need to make any major changes to what she eats or drinks during breastfeeding, though there are a few important considerations to keep in mind.

A Healthy Eating Style is Important for the Mother's Health

One of the amazing characteristics of breast milk is that it can meet the baby's nutritional needs even if the mother is not eating well or is fasting. The fact that the baby won't be harmed by the mother's fasting doesn't mean that the mother won't suffer from the dietary insufficiency. Getting enough vitamins and nutrients is important because the mother needs energy to meet the physical demands of caring for a new baby. During the fasting time, a mother's milk amounts will only change if she is not getting enough calories throughout the entire day and becomes severely dehydrated. According to a study conducted in the United Arab Emirates, there were no significant differences seen in the content of major nutrients of breast milk taken during and after Ramadan. A breastfeeding mother must eat well and rest so that her body can tolerate the demands placed on it while fating. Eating well does not necessarily mean eating more; a mother can think of her breastfeeding time as a continuation of her pregnancy when she ate a well-balanced diet of vegetables, fruit, whole grains, and foods that provide her with protein, iron, and calcium. An occasional treat (dessert) is okay every now and then.

Fasting While Breastfeeding is Fine, But a Mother Should Take It Slow

A breastfeeding mother should take things one day at a time during Ramadan. The age of the baby is very important to take into consideration when fasting. A baby younger than six months is exclusively breastfed and demands more from the mother. An older baby does not feed as often and is easier to take care of. If a mother is feeding and fasting and has no complaints, she should complete her fast for that day; however, if she feels different the next day, she can always stop fasting. As soon as she begins to feel the exhausting pressures of breastfeeding and fasting, such as feeling ill, feeling dizzy, or passing dark yellow urine indicating dehydration, it is okay for her to break her fast and give her kafarah (compensation) for that day. Muslim women who are pregnant or breastfeeding might be exempt from fasting if they feel that the fasting would negatively affect their health or their baby's health. A mother might be expected to make up for the missed fasting at a later time or pay some compensation for not fasting. Consulting a scholar or a book of fiqh is recommended to determine the appropriate guidelines.

Allah's Messenger (may peace be upon him) said, "You must nurse your baby even with your tears," as he recommended Asmaa Bent Abi Bakr (may God be pleased with him) to nurse her baby at the breast!

Scientific research strongly supports the benefits of breastfeeding, and exclusive breastfeeding without introducing any other foods enhances the benefits. WHO/UNICEF reported that the "lack of breastfeeding—and especially lack of exclusive breastfeeding during the first half-year of life—are important risk factors for infant and childhood morbidity and mortality that are only compounded by inappropriate complementary feeding."[166] The impact is lifelong and will affect school performance, productivity, and intellectual and social development.

An example of the lack of knowledge and incorrect beliefs can be seen in an article written in *Okaz* on May 14, 2009. The article was written by Muhammad AlMusbahi about Salih Al Lahidan's opinion about freezing breast-milk in hospitals. Al Lahidan stated that health organizations should not freeze breast-milk and give it to newborns because the milk could be mixed up with milk from other mothers and the child might not know who his milk mother is in the future. Al Lahidan ended his statement by recommending that hospitals use artificial milk, goat's milk, or cow's milk instead of giving the baby human milk that has been donated by a mother who is unknown. This is a clear contradiction to the ayah from Surrat Al Talaq (65:6).

This is 2009, a time when we can use technology to properly label, track, and record donated milk. It is a very easy task to assign specific milk mothers to specific babies. It is even easier to simply document on the infant's official papers that he or she had been given milk by a specific woman. Milk is species specific and human milk is made for human babies and animal milk is made for animal babies.

Breastfeeding and Ecology

Breastfeeding advocacy aims to celebrate women's capacity to sustain life, to cherish the life-giving benefits of breast-milk, and to recognize breastfeeding as the most ecological food system. The positive reasons for a woman to breastfeed are many and include improved health benefits for the mother and child and ensuring the best physical and psychological development of the baby. It is well known that breastfeeding benefits all parts of society: health status, economics, ecological benefits, and social benefits. In my opinion, the least familiar benefit of breastfeeding is the ecological benefit. Breastfeeding is a natural and renewable resource, whereas artificial baby milk (also known as baby formula) is nonrenewable and creates ecological damage at each stage of its production, distribution, and use.

Common sense indicates that breastfeeding protects the environment by reducing the demands made on it and eliminating waste and pollution. Breast milk is a unique food in that its development produces no waste and it causes no pollution. It is also the most energy efficient food production system ever known because it is naturally produced to perfection. The mother's body transforms nutrients from within into a natural, priceless, and specialized food. In contrast, artificial baby milk is produced in factories and converted into powder by exposing the milk to high temperatures. The process uses large amounts of electricity mostly provided by hydroelectric or nuclear power plants worldwide, which is very expensive and definitively has a role in damaging the environment—damaging Mother Earth.

Industrially manufactured, artificial milk goes through many processes, additions, and alterations to convert it from cow's liquid milk to a tin full of powder that infants can ingest. This is why it is confirmed to be vulnerable to contamination by many things, such as bacteria, radioactivity, chemicals, and toxins such as melanin. The media reported that in 2005, the Ministry of Commerce recalled shipments of formula milk that had been delivered to Saudi Arabia from another country because it was contaminated with bacteria that was deadly to infants. This is one example of contamination and an example of the fact that many countries including Saudi Arabia import artificial milk and baby food from other parts of the world. This transportation wastes fuel and contributes to air pollution. The packaging needed for the powdered milk wastes aluminum, plastic, and paper. Feeding the baby artificial milk requires bottles, teats, and other equipment that wastes plastic, rubber, silicon, and glass.

The 550 million tons of artificial milk sold each year to the parents of bottle-fed babies in the United States, when stacked end to end, can circle the earth one and a half times.[157] In Pakistan, the number of feeding bottles sold annually and stacked end to end would reach the top of Mount Everest. Tins, bottles, and all these wastes are not biodegradable and take 200 to 450 years to break down and decompose. To feed a three-month-old baby artificial milk, the mother must prepare one liter of water per day to mix the powder and another two liters to clean and sterilize the bottles and teats. If she is poor and needs wood to make the fire, she would need seventy-three kilograms of wood for one year's worth of sterilizing. In many parts of the world, water and fuel are scarce and not many women are able to keep their bottles and teats clean enough for the babies.[157] Breastfeeding needs no transportation, packing, preparation, or sterilization. It is always available, ready, warm, and sterilized and causes no waste or pollution.

We live in a time where movies like WALL.E seem very close to reality. Our home, our Mother Earth's vitality, is threatened by our continuous destruction and refusal to take care of her. We must begin with our homes and our personal decisions. A mother can contribute to environmental awareness by breastfeeding her baby. The benefits are unmatched.

Birthing Practices

Many mammals show that early contact with their young soon after birth holds an important place in the maintenance of maternal behavior. Increasing evidence indicates that this is also true in humans.[123]

Mary Kroeger, a nurse midwife and lactation specialist, stated the following in her paper prepared for WABA Global Forum II in 2002:

> The partnership of mother and baby is genetically programmed to support the physical, hormonal, and emotional events of pregnancy, labor, birth, and initiation of breastfeeding. The new mother is immediately ready to care for her newborn—to provide warmth, nourishment, and to protect her baby from harm and infection, just as occurred inside her womb. Initiating breastfeeding is easiest and most successful when a mother is physically and psychologically prepared for birth and breastfeeding. (p. 1)

A healthy newborn human is most likely to be separated from his or her mother for sometimes up to days waiting for the mother's milk to come in. During this waiting period, the baby is supplemented by artificial formula unnecessarily. This practice is seen both in traditional and modern settings. This practice is potentially harmful for breastfeeding and ultimately for bonding in the development of the mother-baby relationship.[159] Evidence shows that early touch (within thirty minutes) of the nipple and areola can positively influence this bonding.[153] Birthing methods must be made more humane to allow mothers to put babies to the breast as soon as they are able to, whether the milk comes in or not.

Close observations of ten infants immediately after birth by Windstorm et al.,[153] and observations of thirty-eight infants by Righard and Alade,[121] showed that non-sedated infants follow a predictable pre-feeding behavior pattern. The behavior was seen when the infants were held on the mother's chest immediately after birth, although timing varied widely. The infant's movements begin within twelve to forty-four minutes and spontaneous suckling with good attachment begins at twenty-seven to seventy-one minutes. Sucking movements reached a peak at forty-five minutes and then declined and disappeared by two to two and a half hours post delivery.

Some deliveries can become complicated and the initiation of breastfeeding can be delayed, such as after C-sections. Sometimes the condition of the mother or infant makes the delay of early contact unavoidable, but this must be made the exception and not the rule. C-sections can often be performed with local anesthesia; therefore, breastfeeding can be initiated immediately after birth. If general anesthesia is necessary, breastfeeding can be initiated within just a few hours.[66]

The Global Criteria for the WHO/UNICEF Baby Friendly Hospital Initiative states that mothers in the maternity ward after normal vaginal deliveries should verify that within thirty minutes after birth their babies were given to them to hold with skin to skin contact for at least thirty minutes, and provided help by a staff member to initiate breastfeeding.[165] The Global Criteria also states that at least 50 percent of mothers who delivered by cesarean section should also confirm that within a half hour of being awake and responsive, they were given their babies to hold with skin to skin contact. This statement expresses the strong belief of the importance of initiation of breastfeeding within the first thirty minutes after normal delivery and as soon as possible after C-section. The statement is also supported by a number of research studies conducted over many years.

Righard and Alade performed a study of the effect of early contact on early suckling in 1990 and found a significant difference in the effectiveness of suckling. Comparisons were made of two groups of infants assigned to a contact group or separation group immediately after birth. The first group of thirty infants had immediate contact for at least one hour after birth, which resulted in twenty-four of the babies suckling effectively after a mean of forty-nine minutes. The second group of thirty-four infants had started contact immediately after birth and then were separated for twenty minutes and returned, which resulted in only seven babies sucking correctly.

Four separate studies conducted in the late 1970s and early 1980s showed evidence that early contact resulted in a significant increase in breastfeeding rates at two to three months. The first study was in 1976 by Sosa et al. in Guatemala. Sosa et al. randomly assigned forty women to an early contact group or a control group and then followed up with home visits after three months. The early contact group women were given their babies after delivery of the placenta and episiotomy repair and left together for forty-five minutes. Members of the control group were given their babies twenty-four hours after delivery. The follow-up home visits showed 72 percent of the early contact group continued to breastfeed compared to only 42 percent of the control group. The first group had a mean duration of breastfeeding of 196 days compared to 104 days for the second group.

The second study took place in Sweden. De Chateau and Wiberg studied forty first-time mothers.[50] The moms were randomly assigned to a control group and an intervention group. The intervention consisted of extra contact, which was defined by fifteen to twenty minutes of suckling and skin-to-skin contact during the first hour postpartum. Fifty-eight percent of the mothers in the intervention group were still breastfeeding at three months, whereas only 26 percent of the mothers in the control group were still breastfeeding.

The third study, by Thomson, Hartsock, and Larson,[139] compared the effect of early contact with routine contact in thirty primaparae women who wished to breastfeed. Early contact was initiated within thirty minutes after delivery and continued for up to twenty minutes, and routine contact lasted less than five minutes immediately postpartum and resumed after twelve to twenty-five hours. After two months, nine out of fifteen of the women from the early contact group were breastfeeding without milk supplements compared to only three out of fifteen from the routine contact group.

The fourth research study was conducted in Jamaica and involved comparing two randomly assigned groups. Ali and Lowry compared seventy-two women in two groups: a routine contact group, which started at nine hours postpartum, and an early contact group, which started at forty-five minutes immediately after delivery and then resumed at nine hours.[4] Ali and Lowry found at six weeks postpartum, the rate of exclusive breastfeeding was higher in the early contact group (76%) than in the routine contact group

(49%). After twelve weeks, the early contact group was still showing higher rates (57%) than the routine contact group (27%).

One research study showed that there was a significant effect of early contact after only one week. In 1990, Strachen-Lindenberg, Cabrera, and Jimenez looked at the effect of all early contact, breastfeeding promotion, and rooming-in on both the initiation and continuation of breastfeeding in first-time Nicaraguan mothers.[134] The mothers were randomly assigned to either a control group or an early contact group immediately after birth. In the control group, there was complete separation until discharge, twelve to twenty-four hours post delivery. In the early contact group, mother-infant contact was immediate for forty-five minutes, followed by complete separation until discharge. One week later, the study found that full breastfeeding was significantly higher in the early contact group, but four months afterward, no differences were observed. In this research study, age was not controlled for, although most of the mothers were adolescents.

Perez-Escamilla et al. conducted a meta-analysis of the seven studies mentioned above and found that early contact had a positive effect on the length of time of breastfeeding within three months, but cautioned that the consequence of size across research studies was mixed and that some of the studies involved several other interventions such as breastfeeding guidance and the presence of the father during early contact. These factors might have contributed independently to better the breastfeeding situation.

The use of pain relievers and anesthesia during labor and delivery has been shown in recent studies to contribute to breastfeeding problems. The problems occur because the medications have been found to affect the baby's suckling behavior after birth.[91] So, even if early contact is established, an infant's natural sucking behavior patterns could have been altered in those cases.

A group of mothers studied by Righard and Alade had been administered the analgesic pethidine during labor.[121] Within two hours of delivery, the infants' breastfeeding behavior was observed and they were found to be less likely to suckle correctly or to suckle at all compared to babies born to mothers who had not received pethidine.

Another study by Nissen et al. also compared the breastfeeding behavior of newborns.[105] The group consisted of forty-four babies observed for the first two hours of life. Mothers who did not receive pethidine had infants that showed rooting reflexes earlier and more intensely than those infants born to mothers who had received pethidine. The infants exposed to pethidine (via their mothers) began suckling later. In 1997, Nissen et al. assessed a subsample of thirteen newborns whose mothers had received 100 mg of pethidine. When pethidine was given one to five hours before delivery, suckling behavior was more affected than when it was given eight to ten hours before. A researcher analyzed combined data from a national survey of births in the United Kingdom and a post-questionnaire collected from 1,064 women six weeks after delivery. The results showed 45 percent of women who did not receive pethidine during labor were fully breastfeeding, whereas only 38 percent of the women who did receive pethidine were fully breastfeeding. In 1998, the WHO stated in the book titled *Evidence for the Ten Steps to Successful Breastfeeding*, routine use of pethidine should be kept at a minimum. This is because infants born to mothers who have received pethidine within five hours of delivery are most likely to be depressed and will be delayed in their initiation of breastfeeding.

Alternative approaches of relieving pain during labor and delivery to lessen the side effects to mother and baby are said to be just as effective in pain relief. In 1991, Hofmeyr et al. revealed that severe pain perception was significantly lower in a group of women with companionship (58%) in comparison to a group who had routine care.[76] Kroeger made some suggestions for alternatives to pain medications as methods that serve to reduce mothers' anxiety and fear.[88] In this study, reducing adrenaline was prompted, which in turn lessens the perception of pain.

The issue of integrating humane, nonmedicalized, evidence-based birthing practices as necessary within the work of promoting, protecting, and supporting breastfeeding was emphasized in the workshops at the WABA Global Forum II held in Arusha, Tanzania, September 2002. Since then, WABA has posted a suggested list of Best Practices for Normal Childbirth, which includes the following:

- Care that minimizes routine practices and procedures that are not supported by scientific evidence (e.g., withholding nourishment)
- Care by staff trained in nondrug methods of pain relief

- Supportive policies that encourage mothers and families...[to] hold, breastfeed, and care for their babies

These steps were adapted with permission from the Mother-friendly Childbirth Initiative of the Coalition for Improving Maternity Services and from The Ten Priorities for Perinatal Care.

It is also recommended by the WHO that mothers and infants should not be apart after birth unless there is a medical reason.[159] Ultimately, a baby should be left with its mother from birth onward and allowed to feed from the breast whenever he or she shows signs of readiness. An arbitrary but practical minimum recommendation is for thirty minutes of skin-to-skin contact within the first thirty minutes after birth.

*The following list of references is a list of all the material that was used to write this book and to support the scientific research that went into the study that was conducted in Jeddah, Saudi Arabia.

BIBLIOGRAPHY

1. Al AlSheikh, A. (2006, November 15). How to tackle the diabetes epidemic in Saudi Arabia. *Arab News*. Retrieved March 31, 2007, from http://www.arabnews.com.
2. Al-Daghri, N., Al-Rubean, K., Bartlett, W. A., Al-Attas, O., Jones, A. F., & Kumar S. (2003). Serum leptin is elevated in Saudi Arabian patients with metabolic syndrome and coronary artery disease. *Diabetic Medicine, 20*, 832-837. Retrieved March 1, 2008, from Google Scholar.
3. Al-Hazzaa, H. M. (2007). Pedometer-determined physical activity among obese and non-obese 8- to 12-year-old Saudi schoolboys. *Journal of Physiological Anthropology, 26*, 459-465. Retrieved March 1, 2008, from Google Scholar.
4. Ali, Z., & Lowry, M. (1981). Early maternal-child contact: Effects on later behavior. *Developmental Medicine and Child Neurology, 23*, 337-345.
5. Al-Jassir, M., Moizuddin, S. K., & Al-Bashir, B. (2003). A review of some statistics on breastfeeding in Saudi Arabia. *Nutrition Health, 17*, 123-130. Retrieved March 31, 2007, from ProQuest database.

6. Al-Nozha, M. M., Abdullah, M., Arafah, M. R., Khalil, M. Z., Khan, N. B., Al-Mazrou, Y. Y., et al. (2007). Hypertension in Saudi Arabia. *Saudi Medical Journal, 28,* 77-84. Retrieved March 1, 2008, from Google Scholar.

7. Al-Nozha, M. M., Al-Hazzaa, H. M., Arafah, M. R., Al-Khadra, A., Al-Mazrou, Y. Y., Al-Maatouq, M. A., et al. (2007). Prevalence of physical activity and inactivity among Saudis aged 30-70 years: A population-based cross-sectional study. *Saudi Medical Journal, 28,* 559-568. Retrieved March 1, 2008, from Google Scholar.

8. Al Nuaim, A. R. (2004). Prevalence of glucose intolerance in urban and rural communities in Saudi Arabia. *Diabetic Medicine, 14,* 595-602. Retrieved November 11, 2006, from PubMed database.

9. Al-Othman, A. M., Saeed, A. A., Bani, I. A., & Al-Murshed, K. S. (2002). Mothers' practices during pregnancy, lactation and care of their children in Riyadh, Saudi Arabia. *Saudi Medical Journal, 23,* 909-914. Retrieved November 11, 2006, from ProQuest database.

10. Al Radi, A. O., Ayyub, M., Al Mashat, F. M., Barlas, S. M., Al Hamdan, N. A., Ajarim, D. S., et al. (2000). Primary gastrointestinal cancers in the Western Region of Saudi Arabia. Is the pattern changing? *Saudi Medical Journal, 21,* 730-734. Retrieved May 12, 2007, from PubMed database.

11. Al-Rukban, M. O. (2003). Obesity among Saudi male adolescents in Riyadh, Saudi Arabia. *Saudi Medical Journal, 24,* 27-33. Retrieved March 1, 2008, from Google Scholar.

12. Al-Saeed, W. Y., Al-Dawood, K. M., Bukhari, I. A., & Bahnassy, A. (2007). Prevalence and socioeconomic risk factors of obesity among urban female students in Al-Khobar city, Eastern Saudi Arabia, 2003. *Obesity Reviews, 8*(2), 93-99. Retrieved March 1, 2008, from Google Scholar.

13. Amir, L. H. (2006). International Breastfeeding Journal: Introducing a new journal (Editorial). *International Breastfeeding Journal, 1,* 3. Retrieved February 25, 2008, from http://www.internationalbreastfeedingjournal.com

14. Arenz, S., Rückerl, R., Koletzko, B., & Von Kries, R. (2004). Breastfeeding and childhood obesity: A systematic review. *International Journal of Obesity & Related Metabolic Disorders, 28,* 1247-1256. Retrieved April 6, 2007, from EBSCOhost database.

15. Arnold, L. D. W. (2006). Global health policies that support the use of banked donor human milk: A human rights issue. *International Breastfeeding Journal, 1,* 26. Retrieved February 25, 2008, from http://www.internationalbreastfeedingjournal.com/content/1/1/26.

16. Aspers, P. (2004). Empirical phenomenology. An approach for qualitative research. *Papers in Social Research Methods. Qualitative Series, 9.* Retrieved January 20, 2009.

17. Bailey, C., Pain, R. H., & Aarvold, J. E. (2004). A 'give it a go' breastfeeding culture and early cessation among low-income mothers. *Midwifery, 20,* 240-250.

18. Baker, R. D. (2002). Infant formula safety. *Pediatrics, 110,* 833-835. Retrieved April 6, 2007, from EBSCOhost database.

19. Bandura, A. (1986). *Social foundations of thought and action: A social cognition theory.* Englewood Cliffs, NJ: Prentice-Hall.

20. Beasley, A., & Amir, L. H. (2007). Policy on infant formula industry funding, support or sponsorship of articles submitted for publication. *International Breastfeeding Journal, 2,* 5. Retrieved February 24, 2008, from http://www.internationalbreastfeedingjournal.com/content/2/1/5.

21. Bentley, M. E., Corneli, A. L., Piwoz, E., Moses, A., Nkhoma, J., Carlton Tohill, B., et al. (2005). Perceptions of the role of maternal nutrition in HIV-positive breastfeeding women in Malawai. *The Journal of Nutrition, 135,* 945-949. Retrieved April 20, 2007, from ProQuest database.

22. Bergmann, K. E., Bergmann, R. L., Von Kries, R., Böhm, O., Richter, R., Dudenhausen, J. W., et al. (2003). Early determinants of childhood overweight and adiposity in a birth cohort study: Role of breastfeeding. *International Journal of Obesity, 27,* 162-172. Retrieved March 1, 2008, from Google Scholar.

23. Beshai, J. A. (2008). Are cross-cultural comparisons of norms on death and anxiety valid? *OMEGA, 57*(3), 299-313. Retrieved January 25, 2009 from EBSCOhost database.

24. Betzold, C. M., Laughlin, K. M., & Shi, C. (2007). A family practice breastfeeding education pilot program: An observational, descriptive study. *International Breastfeeding Journal, 2,* 4. Retrieved February 26, 2008, from http://www.internationalbreastfeedingjournal.com/content/2/1/4.

25. Black, R. E., Morris, S. S., & Bryce, J. (2003). Where and why are 10 million children dying every year? *The Lancet, 361,* 2226-2234. Retrieved April 6, 2007, from http://www.thelancet.com.

26. Boeree, C. G. (2006). *Personality theories: Albert Bandura.* Retrieved May 6, 2007, from http://webspace.ship.edu/cgboer/bandura.html.

27. Bortman, M., Brimblecombe, P., & Cunningham, M. A. (2003). Child survival revolution. In *Environmental encyclopedia.* Farmington Hills, MI: Gale Group.

28. Bowen, A. B., & Braden, C. R. (2006). Invasive *enterobacter sakazakii* disease in infants. *Emerging Infectious Diseases, 12,* 1185-1189.

29. Braun-Latour, K. A., & Zaltman, G. (2006). Memory change: An intimate measure of persuasion. *Journal of Advertising Research, 46,* 57-72. Retrieved May 15, 2007, from EBSCOhost database.

30. Breastfeeding is best. (2006). *Population Reports, 33*(4), 12-13. Retrieved March 25, 2007, from EBSCOhost database.

31. Britton, J. R., Britton, H. L., & Gronwaldt, V. (2006). Breastfeeding , sensitivity, and attachment. *Pediatrics, 118*(5), e1436-1443. Retrieved November 10, 2006, from PubMed database.

32. Bronfenbrenner, U. (1979). *The ecology of human development.* Cambridge, MA: Harvard University Press.

33. Bronston, B. (2004, August 2). Nature's own: It's better for baby and cheaper for mom. But there remains among many prospective parents a fundamental lack of awareness about nursing, something the organizers of World Breastfeeding Week are

working to change. *Times-Picayune*, p. 01. Retrieved August 29, 2004, from ProQuest database.

34. Broussard, L. (2006). Understanding qualitative research: A school nurse perspective. *The Journal of School Nursing, 22*(4), 212-218. Retrieved January 25, 2009, from EBSCOhost database.

35. Bystrova, K., Widstrom, A. M., Matthiesen, A., Ransjo-Arvidson, A., Welles-Nystrom, B., Vorontsov, I., et al. (2007). Early lactation performance in primiparous and multiparous women in relation to different maternity home practices: A randomized trial in St. Petersburg. *International Breastfeeding Journal, 2,* 9-22. Retrieved June 9, 2007, from http://www.internationalbreastfeedingjournal. com/content/2/1/9.

36. Chalmers, B. (2001). WHO principles of perinatal care: The essential antenatal, perinatal, and post-partum care course. *Birth, 28,* 202-207.

37. Chalmers, B., & Porter, R. (2001). Assessing effective care in normal labor: The Bologna Score. *Birth, 28*(2), 79-83.

38. Chamblin, C. (2006). Breastfeeding after breast reduction: What nurses & moms need to know. *AWHONN Lifelines, 10,* 42-48. Retrieved May 5, 2007, from EBSCOhost database.

39. Chang, C. T. (2006). Is a picture worth a thousand words? Influence of graphic illustration on framed advertisements. *Advances in Consumer Research, 33,* 104-112. Retrieved May 15, 2007, from EBSCOhost database.

40. Chen, A., & Rogan, W. J. (2004). Breastfeeding and the risk of postneonatal death in the United States. *Pediatrics, 113,* e435-439.

41. Chertok, I. R., & Zimmerman, D. R. (2007). Contraceptive considerations for breastfeeding women within Jewish law. *International Breastfeeding Journal*, *2*, 1. Retrieved February 23, 2008, from http://www.internationalbreastfeedingjournal. com/content/2/1/1.

42. Coalition for Improving Maternity Services. (1996). *Mother-friendly childbirth initiative of the Coalition for Improving Maternity Services*. Retrieved September 23, 2003, from http://www.motherfriendly.org.

43. Coldwell, D. A. L. (2007). Is research that is both causally adequate and adequate on the level of meaning possible or necessary in business research? A critical analysis of some methodological alternatives. *The Electronic Journal of Business Research Methods*, *5*(1), 1-10. Retrieved January 25, 2009 from EBSCOhost database.

44. Colin, W. B., & Scott, J. A. (2002). Breastfeeding: Reasons for starting, reasons for stopping and problems along the way. *Breastfeed Review*, *10*(2), 13-19. Retrieved April 16, 2007, from PubMed database.

45. Collaborative Group on Hormonal Factors in Breast Cancer. (2002). Breast cancer and breastfeeding: Collaborative reanalysis of individual data from 47 epidemiological studies in 30 countries, including 50,302 women with breast cancer and 96,973 women without the disease. *The Lancet*, *360*(9328), 187-195. Retrieved May 5, 2007, from EBSCOhost database.

46. Cooper, D. R., & Schindler, P. S. (2002). *Business research methods* (8th ed.). Boston: Irwin.

47. Creswell, J. W. (2002). *Educational research: Planning, conducting, and evaluating quantitative and qualitative research*. Upper Saddle River, NJ: Pearson.

48. Creswell, J. W. (2005). *Educational research: Planning, conducting, and evaluating quantitative and qualitative research* (2nd ed.). Upper Saddle River, NJ: Merrill Prentice-Hall.

49. Dean, M., & Huitt, W. (1999). *Neighborhood and community.* Retrieved May 5, 2007, from http://chiron.valdosta.edu/whuitt/col/context/neighbor.html

50. De Chateau, P., & Wiberg, B. (1977). Long-term effect on mother-infant behavior of extra contact during the first hour post partum: II. A follow-up at three months. *Acta paediatrica Scandinavica, 66,* 145-151.

51. Denzin, N. K., & Lincoln, Y. S. (2003). *Strategies of qualitative inquiry.* London: Sage.

52. Drudy, D., Mullane, N. R., Quinn, T., Wall, P. G., & Fanning, S. (2006). *Enterobacter sakazakii:* An emerging pathogen in powdered infant formula. *Clinical Infectious Diseases, 42,* 996-1002. Retrieved April 29, 2007, from EBSCOhost database.

53. Edhborg, M., Friberg, M., Lundh, W., & Widström, A. (2005). "Struggling with life": Narratives from women with signs of postpartum depression. *Scandinavian Journal of Public Health, 33,* 261-267. Retrieved March 27, 2008, from Google Scholar.

54. Edmond, K. M., Kirkwood, B. R., Amenga-Etego, S., Owusu-Agyei, S., & Hurt, L. S. (2007). Effect of early infant feeding practices on infection-specific neonatal mortality: An investigation of casual links with observational data from rural Ghana. *The American Journal of Clinical Nutrition, 86,* 1126-1131. Retrieved November 16, 2007, from http://www.ajcn.org.

55. Edmond, K. M., Zandoh, C., Quigley, M. A., Amenga-Etego, S., Owusu-Agyei, S., & Kirkwood, B.

R. (2006). Delayed breastfeeding initiation increases risk of neonatal mortality. *Pediatrics, 117,* e380-386. Retrieved April 21, 2007, from EBSCOhost database.

56. El Hazmi, M. A. F., Warsy, A. S., Al Swailem, A. R., & Al Swailem, A. (1998). Prevalence of hypertension in adult Saudi population. *Saudi Medical Journal, 19,* 117-122. Retrieved November 11, 2006, from http://cat.inist.fr

57. *Enterobacter sakazakii* infections associated with the use of powered infant formula. (2002). *Morbidity & Mortality Weekly Report, 51*(12), 297-301. Retrieved April 29, 2007, from EBSCOhost database.

58. Estrada, B. (2002). Infections associated with powdered infant formula. *Infections in Medicine, 19*(8), 350. Retrieved June 10, 2007, from http://medscape.com.

59. Evans, E. M., Rowe, D. A., Racette, S. B., Ross, K. M., & McAuley, E. (2006). Is the current BMI classification appropriate for black and white postmenopausal women? *International Journal of Obesity, 30,* 837-843. Retrieved June 9, 2007, from EBSCOhost database.

60. Fida, N. M., & Al-Aama, J. Y. (2003). Pattern of infant feeding at a university hospital in western Saudi Arabia. *Saudi Medical Journal, 24,* 725-729. Retrieved November 11, 2006, from ProQuest database.

61. Franks, A., & Ayres, P. (2002). Management issues in healthcare maintaining the quality of medical practice: A system analysis with reference to the training of doctors. *Clinician in Management, 11,* 67-75. Retrieved June 6, 2007, from EBSCOhost database.

62. Ghauri, P., & Grønhaug, K. (2002). *Research methods in business studies: A practical guide* (2nd ed.). Harlow, England: Pearson Education.

63. Giorgi, A. (1979). The relationships among level, type, and structure and their importance for social science theorizing: A dialogue with Shütz. In A. Giorgi, R. Knowles, & D. L. Smith (Eds.), *Duquesne studies in phenomenological psychology* (Vol. 3, pp. 81-92). Pittsburgh, PA: Duquesne University Press.

64. Giugliani, E. R. J. (2004). Common problems during lactation and their management. *Jornal de Pediatria (Rio J), 80*(5 Suppl), S147-S154. Retrieved May 19, 2007, from http://www.scielo.br/pdf/jped/v80n5s0/ en_v80n5s0a06.pdf.

65. Golafshani, N. (2003). Understanding reliability and validity in qualitative research. *The Qualitative Report, 8,* 597-607. Retrieved March 1, 2008, from http://www.nova.edu/ssss/QR/QR8-4/golafshani.pdf.

66. Gonzales, R. B. (1990). A large-scale rooming-in program in a developing country: The Dr. Jose Fabella Memorial Hospital experience. *International Journal of Gynecology and Obstetrics, 31*(Supplement 1), 31-34.

67. Greiner, T., Van Esterik, P., & Latham, M. C. (1981). The insufficient milk syndrome: An alternative explanation. *Medical Anthropology, 5,* 233-260.

68. Groenewald, T. (2004). A phenomenological research design illustrated. International Journal of Qualitative Methods, 3(1). Article 4. Retrieved January 25, 2009 from http://www.ualberta.ca/~iiqm/backissues/3_1/pdf/groenewald.pdf.

69. Grummer-Strawn, L. M., & Zuguo Mei, P. (2004). Does breastfeeding protect against pediatric overweight? Analysis of longitudinal data from the Centers for Disease Control and Prevention Pediatric Nutrition Surveillance System. *Pediatrics, 113*(2), e81-86. Retrieved March 1, 2008, from Google Scholar.

70. Gupta, A., Dadhich, J. P., & Sharma, D. (2006). *Tackling obesity in its infancy* (BPNI Technical Info Series – 8). Retrieved December 11, 2007, from http://www.ifanz-ibfan.org.nz/documents/tackling-obesity-nov'06.pdf.

71. Harder, T., Bergmann, R., Kallischnigg, G., & Plagemann, A. (2005). Duration of breastfeeding and risk of overweight: A meta-analysis. *American Journal of Epidemiology, 162*, 397-403. Retrieved March 1, 2008, from Google Scholar.

72. Hawwas, A. W. (1987). Breastfeeding as seen by Islam. *Popular Science, 7,* 55-58. Retrieved November 10, 2006, from PubMed database.

73. Health Canada. (2005). *Nutrition for healthy term infants: Statement of the Joint Working Group: Canadian Paediatric Society, Dietitians of Canada and Health Canada.* Ottawa, Canada: Minister of Public Works and Government Services. Retrieved June 9, 2007, from http://www.hc-sc.gc.ca/fn-an/pubs/infant-nourrisson/nut_infant_nourrisson_term_e.html.

74. Heimbrook, H. (2005). From data to theory: Elements of methodology in empirical phenomenological research in practical theology. *International Journal of Public Theology, 9*, 273–299. Retreived January 25, 2009 from EBSCOhost database.

75. Hoddinott, P., & Pill, R. (2000). A qualitative study of women's views about how health professionals communicate about infant feeding. *Health Expectations, 3,* 224-233. Retrieved March 27, 2008, from Google scholar.

76. Hofmeyr, G. J., et al. (1991). Companionship to modify the clinical birth environment: Effects on progress and perceptions of labour and breastfeeding. *British Journal of Obstetrics and Gynaecology, 98,* 756-764.

77. Homeier, B. P. (2005, July). *Breastfeeding vs. formula feeding.* Retrieved March 31, 2007, from http://www.kidshealth.org/index.html.

78. Howard, C. R., deBlieck, E. A., Lawrence, R. A., Howard, F. M., Lanphear, B., Oakes, D., et al. (2003). Randomized clinical trial of pacifier use and bottle-feeding or cupfeeding and their effect on breastfeeding. *Pediatrics, 111,* 511-518. Retrieved August 29, 2004, from EBSCOhost database.

79. Huitt, W. (2002). *A systems model of human behavior: The context of development.* Retrieved May 5, 2007, from http://chiron.valdosta.edu/whuitt/materials/systemdlc.html.

80. Huitt, W. (2006). *Educational psychology interactive: Religion.* Retrieved May 5, 2007, from http://chiron.valdosta.edu/whuitt/col/context/religion.html.

81. Ilcol, Y. O., Hizli, Z. B., & Ozkan, T. (2006). Leptin concentration in breast milk and its relationship to duration of lactation and hormonal status. *International Breastfeeding Journal, 1,* 21. Retrieved February 23, 2008, from http://www.internationalbreastfeedingjournal.com/content/1/1/21.

82. *Innocenti declaration 2005: On infant and young child feeding.* (2005). Retrieved March 1, 2008, from http://www.innocenti15.net/declaration.pdf.pdf.

83. Jamal, A. A. (2001). Pattern of breast diseases in a teaching hospital in Jeddah, Saudi Arabia. *Saudi Medical Journal, 22,* 110-113. Retrieved May 12, 2007, from PubMed database.

84. Jones, G., Steketee, R., Black, R., Bhutta, Z., & Morris, S. (2003). How many child deaths can we prevent this year? *The Lancet, 362*(9377), 65-71. Retrieved March 2, 2008, from Google Scholar.

85. Karlsson, G. & Tham, K. (2006). Correlating facts or interpreting meaning: Two different epistemological projects within medical research. *Scandinavian Journal of Occupational Therapy, 13,* 68-75. Retrieved January 25, 2009 from EBSCOhost database.

86. Kendall-Tackett, K. (2007). A new paradigm for depression in new mothers: The central role of inflammation and how breastfeeding and anti-inflammatory treatments protect maternal mental health. *International Breastfeeding Journal, 2,* 6. Retrieved February 25, 2008, from http://www.internationalbreastfeedingjournal.com/content/2/1/6.

87. Knip, M., & Akerblomm, H. K. (2005). Early nutrition and later diabetes risk. *Advances in Experimental Medicine and Biology, 569,* 142-150.

88. Kroeger, M., & Smith, L. (2004). *Impact of birthing practices on breastfeeding.* Boston: Jones and Bartlett.

89. Kroeger, M. (2002). *Birthing practices* (Background paper). Paper presented at the WABA Global Forum II, Arusha, Tanzania.

90. Labbok, M. H. (2001). Effects of breastfeeding on mother. *Pediatric Clinics of North America, 48,* 143-158.

91. La Leche League International. (1997). *The womanly art of breastfeeding* (6th ed.). Schaumberg, IL: Author.

92. Lawrence, R. M., & Lawrence, R. A. (2004). Breastmilk and infection. *Clinics in Perinatology, 31,* 501-528. Retrieved April 21, 2007, from Google Scholar.

93. Mansoor, I. (2001). Profile of female breast lesions in Saudi Arabia. *The Journal of the Pakistan Medical Association, 51*(7), 243-247. Retrieved May 12, 2007, from PubMed database.

94. Mansoor, I., Zahrani, I. H., & Abdul Aziz, S. (2002). Colorectal cancers in Saudi Arabia. *Saudi Medical Journal, 23,* 322-327. Retrieved May 12, 2007, from PubMed database.

95. Marshall, D. C., & Rossman, G. B. (2006). *Designing qualitative research* [Electronic version]. London: Sage. Retrieved September 9, 2007, from Google Scholar.

96. Martin, R. M., Gunnell, D., & Smith, G. D. (2005). Breastfeeding in infancy and blood pressure in later life: Systematic review and meta-analysis. *American Journal of Epidemiology, 161,* 15-26. Retrieved November 11, 2006, from PubMed database.

97. Moore, M. L. (2003). When parents ask...about preterm birth, breastfeeding success, breast cancer, or waterbirth. *Journal of Perinatal Education, 12*(4), 40-43. Retrieved May 5, 2007, from EBSCOhost database.

98. Moore, T., Gauld, R., & Williams, S. (2007). Implementing Baby Friendly Hospital Initiative

policy: The case of New Zealand public hospitals. *International Breastfeeding Journal*, *2*, 8. Retrieved February 25, 2008, from http://www.international-breastfeedingjournal.com/content/2/1/8.

99. Moran, V. H., Dykes, F., Burt, S., & Shuck, C. (2006). Breastfeeding support for adolescent mothers: similarities and differences in the approach of midwives and qualified breastfeeding supporters. *International Breastfeeding Journal*, *1*, 23. Retrieved February 25, 2008, from http://www.international-breastfeedingjournal.com/content/1/1/23.

100. Mortensen, E. L., Michaelsen, K. F., Sanders, S. A., & Reinisch, M. J. (2002). The association between duration of breastfeeding and adult intelligence. JAMA, 287, 2365-2371. Retrieved May 6, 2007, from Google Scholar.

101. Moustakas, C. (1994). *Phenomenological research methods*. London: Sage.

102. Musaiger, A. O. (2004). Overweight and obesity in the Eastern Mediterranean region: Can we control it? *East Mediterranean Health Journal*, *10*, 789-793. Retrieved March 1, 2008, from Google Scholar.

103. Nankunda, J., Tumwine1, J. K., Soltvedt, Å., Semiyaga, N., Ndeezi1, G., & Tylleskär, T. (2006). Community based peer counselors for support of exclusive breastfeeding: Experiences from rural Uganda. *International Breastfeeding Journal*, *1*, 19.Retrieved February 24, 2008, from http://www.internationalbreastfeedingjournal.com/content/1/1/19.

104. Nicoletti, T. A. (2006). Quality of care in evaluating the doctor-patient relationship. *American*

Journal of Bioethics, 6, 44-45. Retrieved June 6, 2007, from EBSCOhost database.

105. Nissen, E., et al. (1995). Effects of maternal pethidine on infants' developing breastfeeding behavior. *Acta Peadiatrica, 84,* 140-145.

106. Nissen, E., et al. (1997). Effects of routinely given pethidine during labour on infants developing breastfeeding behavior. Effects of dose-delivery time interval and various concentrations of pethidine/norpethidine in cord plasma. *Acta peadiatrica, 86,* 201-208.

107. Oddy, W. H., Sly, P. D., de Klerk, N. H., Landau, L. I., Kendall, G. E., Holt, P. G., et al. (2003). Breastfeeding and respiratory morbidity in infancy: A birth cohort study. *Archives of Disease in Childhood, 88,* 224-228. Retrieved March 2, 2008, from Google Scholar.

108. Ogbeide, D. O., Siddiqui, S., Al Khalifa, I. M., & Karim, A. (2004). Breastfeeding in a Saudi Arabian community: Profile of parents and influencing factors. *Saudi Medical Journal, 25,* 580-584. Retrieved March 5, 2006, from ProQuest database.

109. Ogundele, M. O., & Coulter, J. B. S. (2003). HIV transmission through breastfeeding: Problems and prevention. *Annals of Tropical Paediatrics, 23,* 91-106. Retrieved April 20, 2007, from EBSCOhost database.

110. Orne-Gliemann, J., Mukotekwa, T., Perez, F., Miller, A., Sakarovitch, M., Glenshaw, M., et al. (2006). Improved knowledge and practices among end-users of mother-to-child transmission of HIV prevention services in rural Zimbabwe.

Tropical Medicine and International Health, 2, 341-349. Retrieved April 20, 2007, from EBSCOhost database.

111. Owen, C. G., Martin, R. M., Whincup, P. H., Smith, G. D., & Cook, D. G. (2005). Effect of infant feeding on the risk of obesity across the life course: A quantitative review of published evidence. *Pediatrics, 115,* 1367-1377. Retrieved November 11, 2006, from PubMed database.

112. Owen, C. G., Martin, R. M., Whincup, P. H., Smith, G. D., & Cook, D. G. (2006). Does breastfeeding influence risk of type 2 diabetes in later life? A quantitative analysis of published evidence. *American Journal of Clinical Nutrition, 84,* 1043-1054. Retrieved November 11, 2006, from PubMed database.

113. Patton, M. Q. (2002). *Qualitative research & evaluation methods* (3rd ed.). London: Sage.

114. Paley, J. (2005). Phenomenology as rhetoric. *Nursing Inquiry, 12*(2), 106-116. Retrieved January 25, 2009 from EBSCOhost database.

115. Pinhas-Hamiel, O., & Zeitler, P. (2005). The global spread of type-2 diabetes mellitus in children and adolescents. *The Journal of Pediatrics, 146,* 693-700. Retrieved March 1, 2008, from Google Scholar.

116. Piwoz, E. G., & Ross J. S. (2005). Use of population-specific infant mortality rates to inform policy decisions regarding HIV and infant feeding. *The Journal of Nutrition, 135,* 1113-1119. Retrieved June 26, 2007, from Google Scholar.

117. Pugh, L. C., Milligan, R. A., Frick, K. D., Spatz, D., & Bronner, Y. (2002). Breastfeeding duration, costs, and benefits of a support program

for low-income breastfeeding women [Abstract]. *Birth, 29,* 95. Retrieved September 12, 2007, from Google Scholar.

118. Radford, R. (2003). Ban advertising of bottle feeding. *Paediatric Nursing, 15*(10), 4. Retrieved May 15, 2007, from EBSCOhost database. Rajan, L. (1994). The impact of obstetric procedures and analgesia/anesthesia during labour and delivery on breastfeeding. *Midwifery, 10,* 87-103.

119. Rea, M. F., Venâncio, S. I., Batista, L., & Greiner, T. (1999). Determinants of the breastfeeding pattern among working women in São Paulo. *Journal of Human Lactation, 15,* 233-239.

120. Rea, M. F., Venâncio, S. I., Martines, J. C., & Savage, F. (1999). Counselling on breastfeeding: Assessing knowledge and skills. *Bulletin of the World Health Organization, 77,* 492-498. Retrieved September 9, 2007, from Google Scholar.

121. Righard, L., & Alade, M. O. (1990). Effect of delivery room routines on success of first breastfeed. *Lancet, 336*(8723), 1105-1107.

122. Riordan, J. (2005). *Breastfeeding and human lactation* (3rd ed.). Boston: Jones & Bartlett.

123. Rosenblatt, J. S. (1994). Psychology of maternal behavior: contribution to clinical understanding of maternal behavior among human. *Acta Paediatrica Supplement, 397,* 3-8.

124. Sachs, M., Dykes, F., & Carter, B. (2006). Feeding by numbers: An ethnographic study of how breastfeeding women understand their babies' weight charts. *International Breastfeeding Journal, 1,* 29. Retrieved February 24, 2008, from http://

www.internationalbreastfeedingjournal.com/content/1/1/29.

125. Sadauskait-Kuehne, V., Ludvigsson, J., Padaiga, Ž., Jašinskien, E., & Samuelsson, U. (2004). Longer breastfeeding is an independent protective factor against development of type 1 diabetes mellitus in childhood. *Diabetes/Metabolism Research and Reviews, 20,* 150-157.

126. Schiff, L. (2006). Breastfeeding makes for better health. *Mount Sinai Journal of Medicine, 73,* 571-572. Retrieved April 6, 2007, from EBSCOhost database.

127. Seidman, I. (2006). *Interviewing as qualitative research: A guide for researchers in education and the social sciences* (3rd ed.). New York: Teachers College Press.

128. Shaffer, D. R. (1993). *Developmental psychology: Childhood and adolescence* (3rd ed.). Pacific Grove, CA: Brooks/Cole.

129. Shawky, S., & Abalkhail, B. A. (2003). Maternal factors associated with the duration of breastfeeding in Jeddah, Saudi Arabia. *Paediatric Perinatal Epidemiology, 17,* 91-96. Retrieved March 5, 2006, from ProQuest database.

130. Shirima, R., Greiner, T., Kylberg, E., & Gebre-Medhin, M. (2000). Exclusive breastfeeding is rarely practiced in rural and urban Morogoro, Tanzania. *Public Health Nutrition, 4,* 147-154. Retrieved April 20, 2007, from Google Scholar.

131. Sikorski, J., Renfrew, M. J., Pindoria, S., & Wade, A. (2003) Support for breastfeeding mothers: A systematic review. *Paediatric and Perinatal*

Epidemiology, 17, 407-417. Retrieved March 1, 2008, from Google Scholar.

132. Smith, J. (2003). *Qualitative psychology: A practical guide to research methods.* New York: Sage.

133. Sosa, R., et al. (1976). *The effect of early mother-infant contact on breastfeeding, infection and growth.* (Ciba Foundation Symposium No.45 (new series): Breastfeeding and the mother). Amsterdam, the Netherlands: Elsevier.

134. Stratechen-Lindenberg, C., Cabrera-Artola, R., & Jimenez, V. (1990). The effect of early post-partum mother-infant contact and breastfeeding promotion on the incidence and continuation of breastfeeding. *International Journal of Nursing Studies, 27*(3), 179-186.

135. Stuebe, A. M., Rich-Edwards, J. W., Willett, W. C., Manson, J. E., & Michels, K. B. (2005). Duration of lactation and incidence of type 2 diabetes. *JAMA, 294,* 2601- 2610.

136. Szajewska, H., Horvath, A., Koletzko, B., & Kalisz, M. (2006). Effects of brief exposure to water, breast-milk substitutes, or other liquids on the success and duration of breastfeeding: A systematic review. *Acta Pædiatrica, 95,* 145-152. Retrieved March 22, 2007, from EBSCOhost database.

137. Taha, T., Kumwenda, N. I., Hoover, D. R., Kafulafula, G., Fiscus, S. A., Nkhoma, C., et al. (2006). The impact of breastfeeding on the health of HIV-positive mothers and their children in sub-Saharan Africa. *Bulletin of the World Health Organization, 84,* 546-554. Retrieved April 20, 2007, from EBSCOhost database.

138. Taveras, E. M., Li, R., Grummer-Strawn, L., Richardson, M., Marshal, R., Rego, V. H., et al. (2004). Opinions and practices of clinicians associated with continuation of exclusive breastfeeding. *Pediatrics, 113*(4), e283-290. Retrieved August 29, 2004, from EBSCOhost database.

139. Thomson, M. E., Hartsock, T. G., & Larson, C. (1979). The importance of immediate postnatal contact: Its effect on breastfeeding. *Canadian Family Physician, 25,* 1374-1378.

140. Torqus, J., & Gotsch, G. (2004). *The womanly art of breastfeeding* (7th ed.). Shaumburg, IL: La Leche League International.

141. Torvaldsen, S., Roberts, C. L., Simpson, J. M., Thompson, J. F., & Ellwood, D. A. (2006). Intrapartum epidural analgesia and breastfeeding: A prospective cohort study. *International Breastfeeding Journal, 1,* 24. Retrieved February 24, 2007, from http://www.internationalbreastfeedingjournal.com/content/1/1/24.

142. United Nations Children's Fund. (n.d.). *Infant and young child feeding and care.* Retrieved March 10, 2006, from http://www.unicef.org/nutrition/index_breastfeeding.html.

143. Ursin, G., Bernstein, L., Lord, S. J., Karim, R., Deapen, D., Press, M. F., et al. (2005). Reproductive factors and subtypes of breast cancer defined by hormone receptor and histology. *British Journal of Cancer, 93,* 364-371. Retrieved May 5, 2007, from EBSCOhost database.

144. Van Den Hazel, P., Zuurbier, M., Babisch, W., Bartonova, A., Bistrup, M. L., Bolte, G., et al.

(2006). Today's epidemics in children: Possible relations to environmental pollution and suggested preventive measures. *Acta Pædiatrica, 95,* 18-25. Retrieved May 5, 2007, from EBSCOhost database.

145. van Kaam, A. (1966). *Existential foundations of psychology.* Pittsburgh, PA: Duquesne University Press.

146. van Manen, M. (2002). *Phenomenological Inquiry.* Retrieved January 20, 2009 from http://www.phenomenologyonline.com/inquiry/1.html.

147. von Eckartsberg, R. (1986). *Life-world experience: Existential-phenomenological research approaches to psychology.* Washington, DC: Center for Advanced Research in Phenomenology & University Press of America.

148. Walker, M. (2002). *Core curriculum for lactation consultant practice.* Sudbury, MA: Jones & Bartlett.

149. Weinberg, G. (2000). The dilemma of postnatal mother-to child transmission of HIV: To breast-feed or not? *Birth, 27*(3), 199-205. Retrieved April 21, 2007, from EBSCOhost database.

150. Westdahl, C., & Page-Goertz, S. (2006). Promotion of breastfeeding: Beyond the benefits. *International Journal of Childbirth Education, 21*(4), 8-16. Retrieved March 22, 2007, from EBSCOhost database.

151. Williams, H. G. (2006). And not a drop to drink: Why water is harmful for newborns. *Breastfeeding Review, 14*(2), 5-9.

152. Win, N. N., Binns, C. W., Zhao, Y., Scott, J. A., & Oddy, W. H. (2006). Breastfeeding duration in

mothers who express breast milk: A cohort study. *International Breastfeeding Journal, 1*, 28. Retrieved February 23, 2007, from http://www.internationalbreastfeedingjournal.com/content/1/1/28.

153. Widstrom, A-M., et al. (1987). Gastric suction in healthy newborn infants. *Acta Paediatrica Scandanavica, 76*, 566-572.

154. Widstrom, A-M., et al. (1990). Short-term effects of early suckling and touch of the nipple on maternal behavior. *Early Human Development, 21*, 153-163.

155. Wolcott, H. F. (2001). *Writing up qualitative research* (2nd ed.). London: Sage.

156. Wolf, J. H. (2003). Low breastfeeding rates and public health in the United States. *American Journal of Public Health, 93*, 2000-2010. Retrieved August 29, 2004, from EBSCOhost database.

157. World Alliance for Breastfeeding Action. (1997). *Breastfeeding nature's way.* Retrievedfrom http://www.waba.org.

158. World Health Organization. (1992). *The global criteria for the WHO/UNICEF Baby Friendly Hospital Initiative.* Geneva, Switzerland: WHO/UNICEF.

159. World Health Organization. (1998). *Evidence for the ten steps to successful breastfeeding.* Geneva, Switzerland: Author.

160. World Health Organization. (2001, January). *The ten priorities for perinatal care.* Presented at the WHO-Euro Child Health and Development Unit, Bologna Perinatal Task Force Meeting.

161. World Health Organization. (1998). *Child health and development: Evidence for the ten steps of successful breastfeeding* (Revised). Geneva, Switzerland: Author.

162. World Health Organization. (2001). *The optimal duration of exclusive breastfeeding. Report of an expert consultation.* Geneva, Switzerland: World Health Organization Department of Nutrition and Health Development. Retrieved July 9, 2007, from http://www.who.int/child-adolescenthealth/New_Publications/NUTRITION/WHO_CAH_01_24.pdf.

163. World Health Organization. (2002). *The optimal duration of exclusive breastfeeding, results of a WHO systematic review* (WHO Note for the Press, No. 7.2). Geneva, Switzerland: Author.

164. World Health Organization. (2004). *Child and adolescent health and development.* Retrieved March 22, 2007, from http://www.who.int/child-adolescenthealth/ NUTRITION/infant_exclusive.htm.

165. World Health Organization/United Nations Children's Fund. (1992). *International child health: A collaborative study on breastfeeding.* Geneva, Switzerland: World Health Organization.

166. World Health Organization/United Nations Children's Fund. (2004). *WHO library cataloguing-in-publication data. Global strategy for infant and young child feeding.* Retrieved March 5, 2006, from http://www.who.int/child-adolescenthealth/ NUTRITION/global_strategy.htm.

167. Wright, A. L., Bauer, M., Naylor, A., Sutcliffe, E., & Clark, L. (1997). Increasing breastfeeding rates to reduce infant illness at the community level. *Pediatrics, 10,* 837-844. Retrieved August 5, 2006, from http://pediatrics.aappublications.org/cgi/content/abstract/101/5/837.

168. Xu, F., Liu, X., Binns, C. W., Xiao, C., Wu, J., & Lee, A. H. (2006). A decade of change in breast-feeding in China's far north-west. *International Breastfeeding Journal, 1,* 22. Retrieved February 25, 2008, from http://www.internationalbreastfeed-ingjournal.com/content/1/1/22.

Made in the USA
Charleston, SC
18 August 2010